TAI CHI

CHRISTIAN F. HANCHE

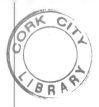

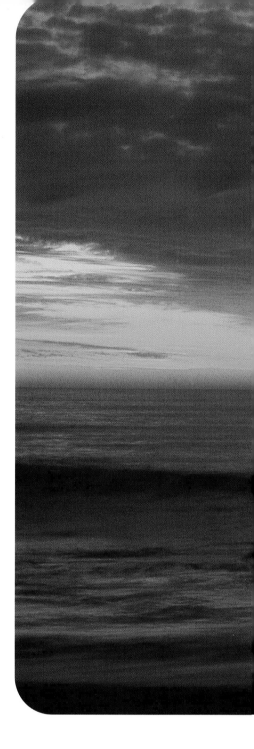

First published in 2002 by
New Holland Publishers
London • Cape Town • Sydney • Auckland

86 Edgware Road
London W2 2EA
United Kingdom

80 McKenzie Street
Cape Town 8001
South Africa

14 Aquatic Drive
Frenchs Forest, NSW 2086
Australia

218 Lake Road
Northcote, Auckland
New Zealand

ISBN 1 84330 002 8 (HB)
ISBN 1 85974 997 6 (PB)

Publisher: Mariëlle Renssen
Managing Editors: Claudia Dos Santos, Mari Roberts
Managing Art Editor: Peter Bosman
Editor: Gill Gordon
Designer: Sheryl Buckley
Illustrator: Alzette Prins
Production: Myrna Collins

Consultant: Harry Cook

Reproduction by Hirt & Carter (Cape) Pty Ltd
Printed and bound in Singapore by Craft Print International Ltd

2 4 6 8 10 9 7 5 3 1

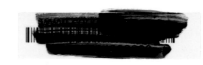

TAI CHI

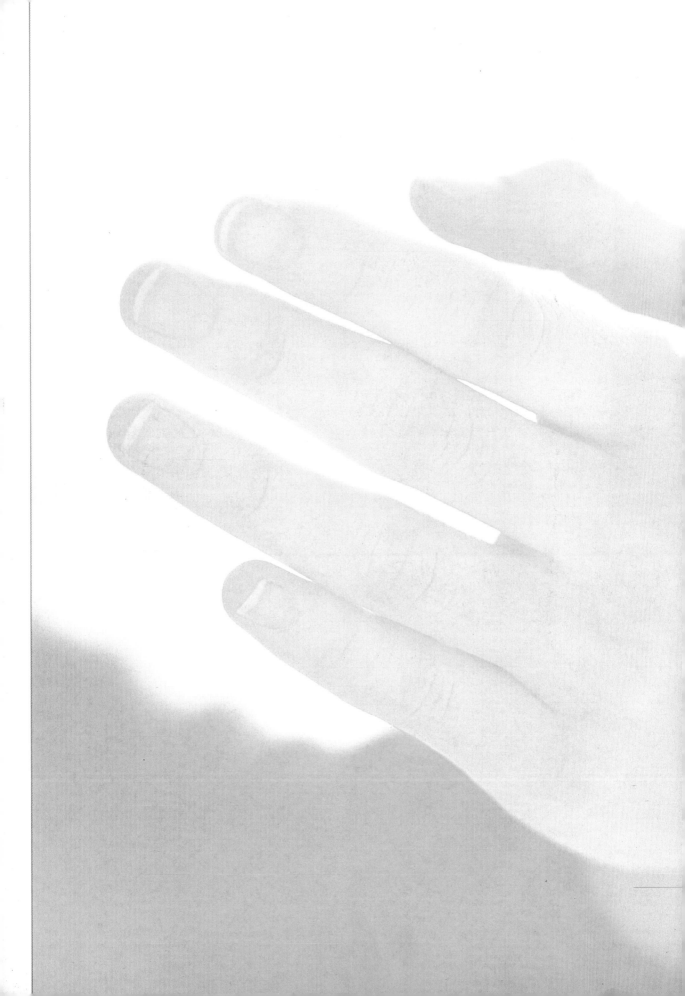

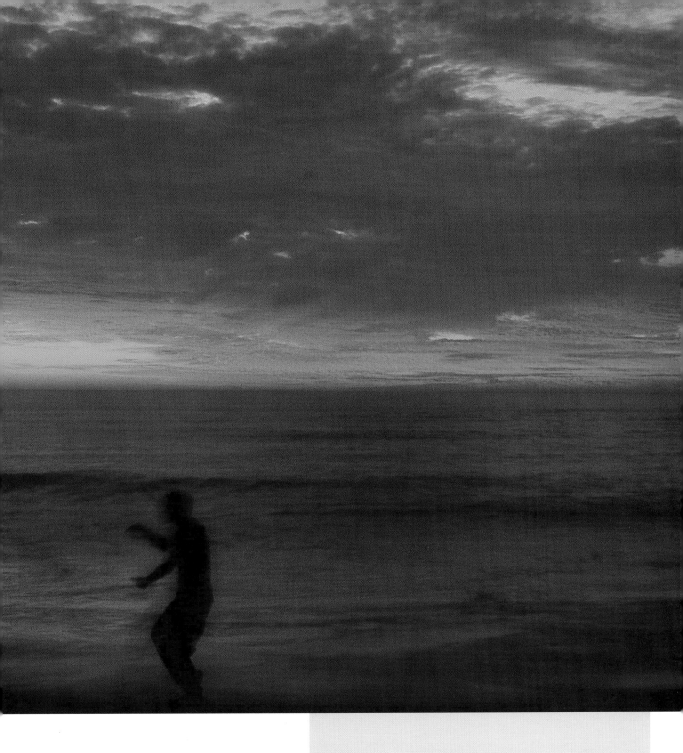

DEDICATED TO:

My parents;
Sifu Derek Frearson for his dedication and commitment;
Sifu Leslie Reed for his tutelage and adherance to
tradition; Sifu Marco Kavalieratos for his generosity
of spirit; W.O.1 - J.H.N. Roodman (retired) for the truest
ideals of leadership.

C O N T E N T S

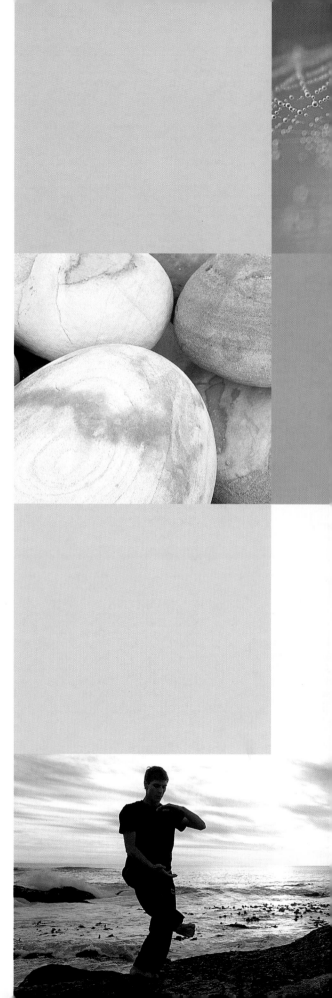

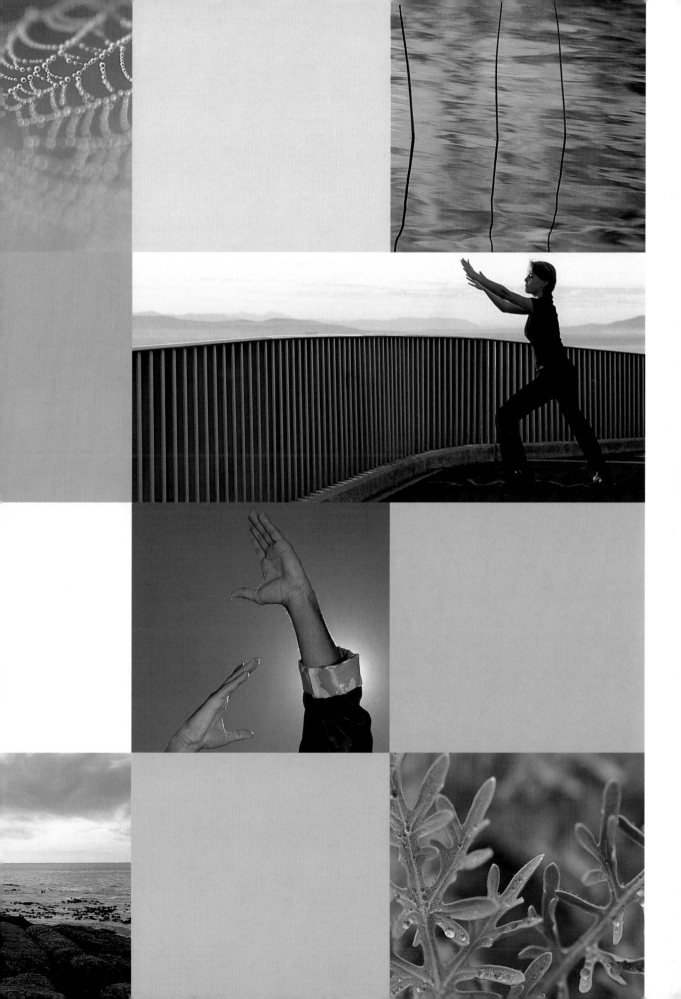

INTRODUCTION

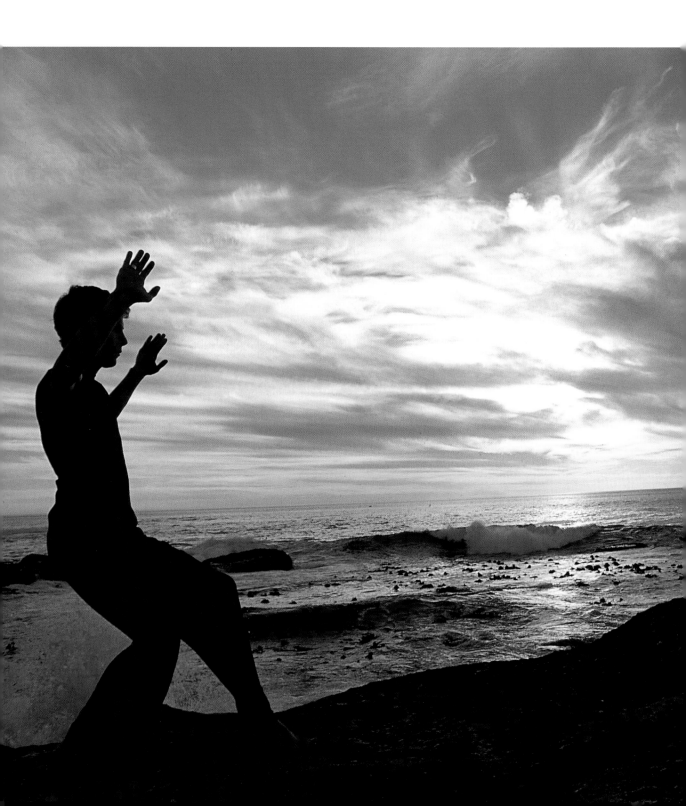

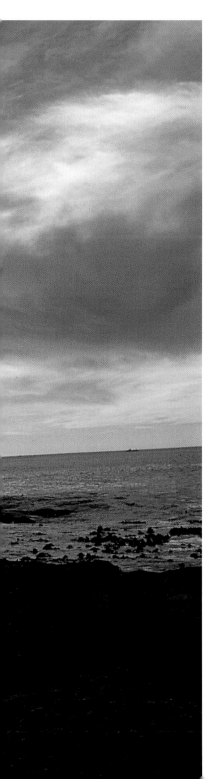

TAI CHI CHUAN, *which translates literally to mean 'Supreme Ultimate Fist', is a martial art of Chinese origins. Like the Tao, the symbol representing Yin and Yang, there exists within the art a dynamic duality. While the martial aspect emphasizes locks, blocks, punches and kicks, there are also movements that promote stretching, strength, flexibility and relaxation. Each aspect has some qualities of the other – they cannot exist apart. To view only one aspect of the art represents a loss of substance, without which you are left with a set of movements which have no meaning or purpose.*

The techniques and movements that are learned in Tai Chi Chuan nowadays are often mere shadows of the originals. However, even though we have progressed far past the days of facing each other in hand to hand combat, it is important that we remain in touch with the origins of Tai Chi, not to encourage the original martial intent behind the art, but to honour the history and traditions of the movements.

For centuries, the Chinese studied the human body in order to better understand the ailments that afflict it. Through careful research and meticulous observation, they formulated various exercises and breathing methods to promote health and vitality. These were gradually incorporated into the various Martial Arts of China, forming the basis of movements which are widely practised throughout the world today.

Tai Chi Chuan unites physical motion with mental focus and concentration. The meditative nature and tranquillity of the movements, combined with deep breathing, benefits the internal organs of the body. Due to the nature of the exercises, age and fitness are not limiting factors, and Tai Chi can be practised safely by people who are often unable to participate in other sporting activities due to physical limitations.

Left **The meditative, tranquil nature of Tai Chi represents one part of its intrinsic dualism. The 'harder' martial arts aspect represents the other side.**

Thirty spokes share the wheel's hub,
It is the centre hole that
makes it useful.
Shape clay into a vessel,
It is the space within that
makes it useful.
Cut doors and windows for a room,
It is the holes which make it useful.
Therefore benefit comes
from what is there,
usefulness from what is not.

Lao Tzu

The Taoist has no ambition, therefore
he can never fail.
He who never fails always succeeds.
He who always succeeds
is all-powerful.

Unknown

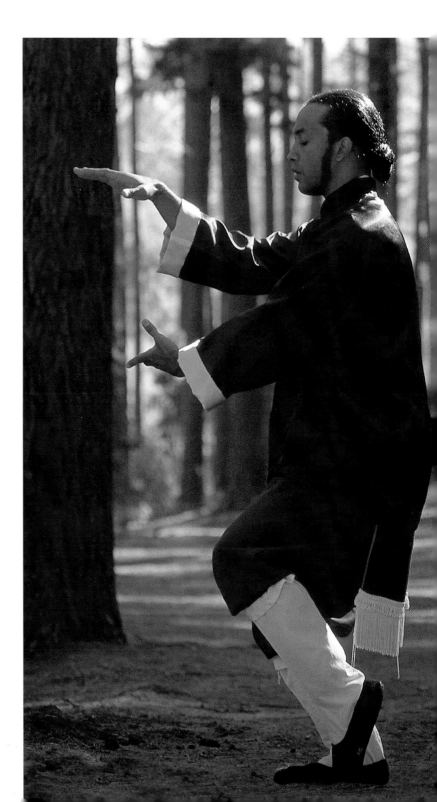

ORIGINS & TRADITIONS

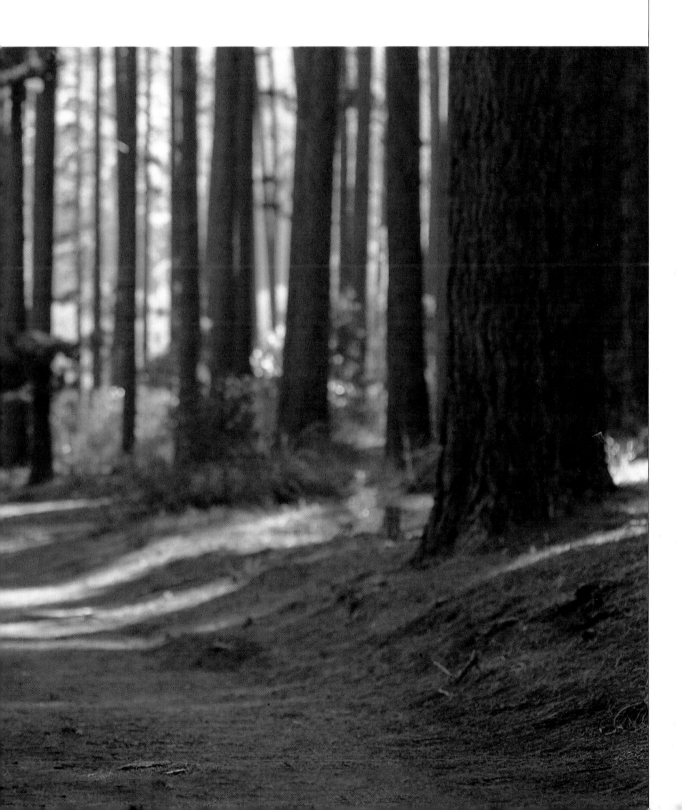

HISTORY & BACKGROUND

MYTHS and legends abound about the origins of the martial arts in China, which, for hundreds of years, were taught in relative, if not total, secrecy by masters of these arts. Prospective students often had to do many months of menial chores on behalf of the Master before being admitted as a student. On admittance, students swore an oath not to reveal the teachings of the art to anybody outside the school, a tradition that still exists in some martial arts schools.

The masters would sometimes withhold an aspect of their art from most of their students, picking just one or two students to whom they would teach the entire style. Sometimes a master would die before he could do this, and so aspects of an art would be lost. Neither masters nor students kept written records, and therefore as the history and training were passed on to each new generation of students through word of mouth, styles inevitably came to differ through the passage of time.

The original thoughts behind the Martial Arts in China derive from three main philosophies.

The first is Confucianism. Founded in c500BC and based on the teachings of Confucius, it deals with people and their place in society, with reverence for traditions and family ancestors.

The second philosophy is Taoism, which is founded on the teachings of Lao Tzu (born c600BC).

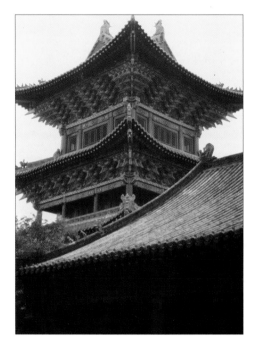

Taoism looks at life and the universe as having an ordered balance and unity. Although many of the concepts ascribed to Lao Tzu predate him by a few thousand years, he is still considered the founder of Taoism.

The third philosophy is Buddhism, founded in c530BC by Prince Gautama Siddhartha of India, whose adherents seek spiritual enlightenment through meditation and contemplation.

Buddhism was introduced via the trade routes from India and quickly took root all over China. One of the forms of Buddhism that came to be practised in China is known as Ch'an Buddhism. Various temples were built, of which the most famous is the Shaolin Temple, set in the foothills of the Songshan Mountains of central China. Built about AD495, the Shaolin Temple quickly became the centre for religious studies in that part of China.

Some 80 years later, an Indian monk, Bodhidharma (known to the Chinese as Ta-Mo), arrived at the Temple. Noticing that the monks were suffering physically from the long hours of meditation, Bodhidharma took it upon himself to improve the situation. Combining breathing techniques with physical movements, and adding these to indigenous Chinese fighting arts, he formulated a number of physical routines based largely on the observed movements of certain animals. These became the foundation for Shaolin Chuan (called Shaolin boxing or Kung Fu in the West).

Above **At the height of its power, the Shaolin Temple housed 1500 monks, 500 of whom were 'fighting' monks.**

Although the Songshan Shaolin Temple is the most famous, recent discoveries in China have revealed the possible existence in the southern parts of China of one, if not two, other temples which were named Shaolin.

Unfortunately, 1500 years of internal strife between various warlords and their armies has left almost no written or physical proof of the exact locations of these temples. However their existence probably accounts for the two distinct systems that exist within Shaolin Kung Fu: the Northern, which emphasizes long low stances and big flowing arm movements; and the Southern, with shorter erect stances and the emphasis on smaller arm movements.

Unlike the West, where differences in religion shut people off from one another, in ancient China, Buddhists, Confucianists and Taoists studied in the same institutions and visited each others' places of worship. Temples were often the only places of learning and monks would travel to another temple to study a particular subject or art.

A 12th-century Taoist monk, Chang San-feng, who was reputed to be a Master of Shaolin Kung Fu, is credited

Above **A fight between a snake and a crane provided the inspiration for the philosophy behind Tai Chi Chuan.**

with being the founder of Tai Chi Chuan. After years of extensive travel and study he returned to the Taoist monastery in the Wu Tang mountains where he took up a life of meditation and contemplation.

Legend has it that Chang San-feng was meditating outdoors one day when he was disturbed by the sounds

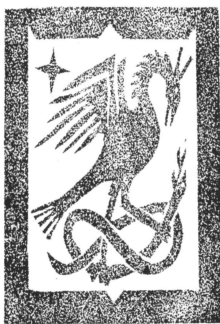

of a fight between a snake and a crane, so he settled down to watch. The crane stabbed at the snake with its beak, the snake twisted away and struck at the crane, which brushed the snake aside with its wing. The snake kept attacking and was repulsed by the crane, the crane's attacks being dissolved by the snake's twisting and coiling. This went on and on, with neither managing to overwhelm the

other, until they eventually tired and went their separate ways. Chang San-feng realized he had witnessed the living embodiment of a Taoist saying *'the strong becomes yielding, while the yielding becomes strong'.*

Understanding the value of softness and yielding in the face of an attack, and using his knowledge of martial arts, Chang San-feng formulated a system which became the basis for a new train of thought in the Martial Arts of China. He subsequently opened what became known as the Wu Tang school of 'soft arts'. As a result, there are two main schools of thought running through the Martial Arts of China. The 'hard' school with its roots in Shaolin traditions, and the 'soft' school with its roots in the Wu Tang mountains.

After this, the history of Tai Chi Chuan becomes unclear, due to a lack of documented facts. What facts do exist tend to be conflicting and vague, but the story picks up again in the 1600s with Ch'en Wang Ting *(see page 17)*, and follows a reasonably clear line through to the founder of the Yang style of Tai Chi Chuan, Yang Lu Chuan (1799–1872). The communist takeover of mainland China in 1949 resulted in a flood of refugees to the West, bringing their culture and traditions, one of which is the ancient art of Tai Chi Chuan.

PHILOSOPHY

TWO of the three philosophies that affected life in early China had a large influence on the development of the Martial Arts in China. These were Buddhism and Taoism (pronounced 'dowism'), and most of the Martial Arts styles were founded in temples practising one or other philosophy.

Due to the Shaolin Temple being Buddhist, most 'hard' styles (those rooted in the Shaolin tradition), have an underlying Buddhist philosophy. The 'soft' schools (which originated in the Wu Tang mountains), convey the teachings and thoughts of Taoism. We can only generalize this in a broad sense because there has been so much integration of these two philosophies within the Chinese Martial Arts that nowadays most styles embody aspects of both schools.

The Yin Yang symbol, which represents the duality of life and of the universe, is Taoist. In the West, it has become an almost universal symbol associated with the schools of Chinese Martial Arts. In contrast, nearly every martial arts school in the East has a painting or mural of the Buddhist monk, Ta-Mo.

Lao Tzu, the founder of Taoism, was born in a peasant village in Hunan province in 604BC. His family name was Li and his proper name Erh, but

other than that, very little is known of his life, other than that, at some point, he was appointed to the position of *Shih* at the royal court of the Chou dynasty (c1111–255BC).

Today, a *Shih* is an historian, but in ancient China, the *Shih* were scholars who specialized in the study of divination and astrology, and were charged with the safekeeping of the sacred books. It was in the role of *Shih* that the title *'Lao Tzu'*, meaning 'Old Sage', was awarded. This also explains why many of the concepts and ideas he wrote about predate him.

It is said that, during his time at the royal court, Lao Tzu met Confucius and they had a discussion on the ethical teachings of the ancient philosophers. Confucius was so astounded by what Lao Tzu said to him, that he didn't utter a word for three days afterwards.

Legend has it that, tired of his life in the royal court, Lao Tzu decided to travel westward. Upon reaching the western limits of the kingdom, he was stopped by the gatekeeper of the western pass. The gatekeeper asked Lao Tzu to write down some thoughts

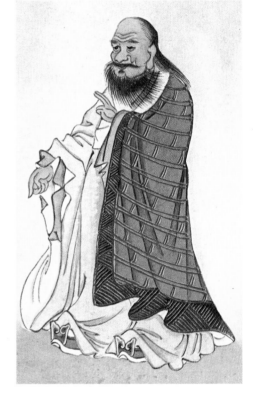

for him before travelling on. Lao Tzu obliged, and it is these writings that became known as the *Tao-te Ching*.

The book, written in two parts and consisting of just 5000 characters, are his ideas of the Tao or 'Way' (also known as the Supreme Principle), with its central theme of 'te' or virtue.

Lao Tzu then continued westward and disappeared into the wilderness of what is now Tibet.

Top **Lao Tzu, the founder of Taoism, was a Shih, or scholar. His writings form the basis of the Tao, or 'Way'.**

In Chinese history, there are many notable men who performed some great deed or deeds, only to disappear into obscurity. Luckily, some leave behind them a legacy and, in this case, the legacy was the basis for Taoism.

Taoism is the fundamental belief that the universe is balanced by the harmonious interaction of opposites.

If there is hard, there must be soft; rigidity then suppleness; light then darkness; Yin then Yang. These opposites connect and change from one to the other with constant movement and harmony, forming a balanced whole. Any imbalance causes disharmony and interrupts the natural flow of change from one to the other. The sages believed that to achieve this balance is to be one with life, nature and the universe, not separate from it.

The early Taoist sages led relatively simple lifestyles, spending much of their time observing and studying their immediate environment. They looked closely at man's interaction with nature and tried to formulate ways and ideals that would allow him to live in harmony with the natural world around him.

Through study they came to understand the importance of maintaining a balanced lifestyle. By combining diet

Right **As water nourishes and sustains a plant, balance and harmony are essential for healthy personal growth.**

and exercise, they realized this would lead to longer, healthier lives. The idea of living longer fascinated them, and they became almost obsessive in their studies of life and longevity. There are many legends of Taoist sages who lived for a hundred years or more.

From its inception, Taoist ideas have permeated Chinese culture, art and philosophy. Rulers have governed by them, artists have depicted Taoist concepts, and poets have written reams that incorporate Taoist principles.

In Taoism, there are no prayers to give or be answered, no sacrifices to be made, no trappings of religion. The Tao simply *is*. Nevertheless, religious Taoism took root and today there are temples and shrines all over China, with priests, prayers and everything that comes with organized religious beliefs. Most early religious Taoism centred on astrology, alchemy and immortality, with a healthy regard for

sexual practices and the 'correct' way to have sex in order to preserve and balance energies and emotions within the physical body.

Taoism is a philosophy of life and of how to achieve balance in life. It is not based on faith in an intangible deity. Taoism does not have an all-powerful figurehead. It looks at man as the microcosm and at how he interacts with his universe, or macrocosm.

Although Taoism originated in China, it is timeless in its theory. It is neither cultural nor regional, it is universal. There are no prejudices, no racial conflicts or class distinction. It is a living belief in a set of principles that allows man to bring balance and harmony into his life, and balance to the universe in which he exists.

In the end, it is up to each individual to find his or her own way, to reach a balance within their lives, and in so doing find their 'Tao'.

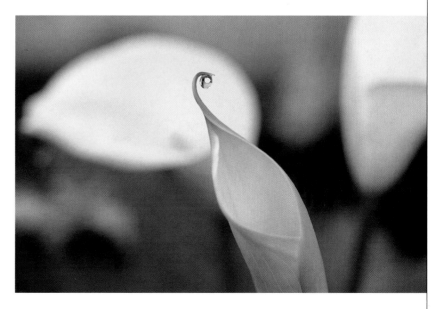

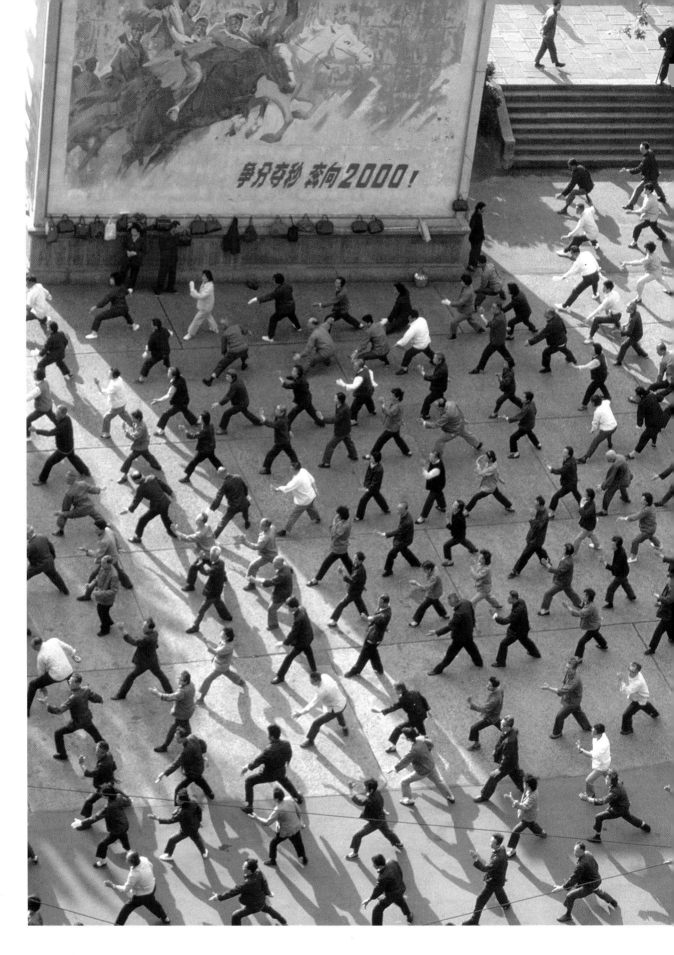

争分夺秒 奔向2000！

STYLES

THROUGHOUT the long history of Chinese Martial Arts, there have been many styles. Some have come and gone, while others remain. The number that have been lost will never be known and, of those that remain, many will probably never be seen outside China.

Through the years, changes in style were inevitable. Styles were sometimes combined, or were shortened or modified to incorporate new ideas or techniques. Changes also came about due to circumstances, such as the uniting of families through marriage.

Many styles became known as 'family' styles or systems. An ancestor may have been a great teacher or may have been the last, or only, student of some Master. Out of respect for the ancestor or Master, the student would decide not to pass on his knowledge to anyone outside the immediate family. This stipulation sometimes remained for many generations.

Meanwhile, changes within a style would take place through the course of the years. A family might be killed outright by a natural disaster such as a flood or earthquake, or the village

Left **Throughout China, it is common for people to gather outdoors to perform their daily Tai Chi exercises.**

might be overrun by a warlord, with everyone put to death. Circumstances such as these could mean the loss of an entire style.

Sometimes styles were united by marriage and parents would then teach their children the combined family system. Women were not precluded from training and a number of women became famous as martial arts practitioners. For instance, Yim Wing Chun, the founder of Wing Chun Kung Fu, was initially trained by a famous Buddhist nun, Ng Mui.

The history of Tai Chi Chuan is no different from that of other Chinese martial arts in its lack of written records. After Chang San-feng *(see page 13)*, there is a large gap, but eventually Tai Chi Chuan became a 'family' system and to this day the styles carry the family names of their founders. The five main styles are Chen, Yang, Wu (or Hao), Wu and Sun.

Chen is considered to be the oldest style and the starting point from which the others developed. Named for its founder, Ch'en Wang Ting (1597 –1664), it remained a closely guarded secret within the Chen family village for many years. Only select members of the family were taught the style and no outsiders were permitted to participate in the training.

Roughly two hundred years later, a young man, Yang Lu Chuan (1799–1872) became the first outsider to be taught the Chen style. Accounts vary as to how and why he was accepted, but he became the founder of the Yang style. Yang Lu Chuan was renowned as a master of his art and even travelled to Beijing where he taught at the Imperial Court.

The Wu (Hao) style was founded by Wu Yu Hsiang (1812–1880), a student of Yang Lu Chuan. He studied the Chen style as well, and combined the two into the Wu (Hao) style. Wu Yu Hsiang taught his version of the art to his nephew and he, in turn, passed it on to Hao Wei Chen, who made a large contribution to the art. As a result, this style is sometimes referred to as the Hao style.

The Wu style was founded by Wu Chuan Yu (1834–1902), yet another student of Yang Lu Chuan, who apparently worked at the Imperial Palace as a bodyguard.

The youngest style is the Sun style, founded by Sun Lu Tang (1860–1932), a student of Hao Wei Chen, who combined his knowledge of Tai Chi Chuan with his knowledge of Hsing-I and Ba Kua to formulate his own style.

The most popular style practised outside China is the Yang style.

UNIFORMS, WEAPONS & GRADING

TRADITIONAL Tai Chi uniforms were simple and practical. They were neither flashy nor gaudy in colour and were rather plain in cut and style. Parts of the uniform were often worn as normal daily clothing and not specifically for practising Tai Chi. In China nowadays, most people train in tracksuits and trainers, or any other loose, comfortable clothing. It is only in the West that a formal uniform is worn for Tai Chi training. You should discuss uniform with your instructor.

PANTS

Pants were traditionally made from a rough homespun fabric, with a draw-string tie at the waist. Some also had draw-strings at the bottom of each leg. Generally, pants were held up by a sash wound around the waist. Modern pants have retained the same cut, with the traditional draw-strings replaced by elastic at the waist and legs.

Although cotton is still the most commonly used fabric, satin or silk pants (and jackets) are also available.

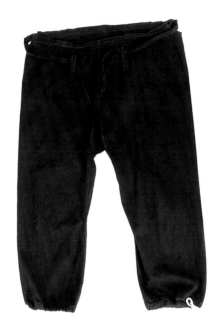

JACKETS

Traditional jackets are made from cotton and are sometimes slightly padded to provide insulation against the weather. The jacket is normally worn over a light T-shirt or some form of undergarment.

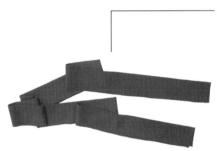

SASH

Traditionally, a two- to three-metre-long sash was wound around the waist a number of times before being tied or tucked in. The sash was sometimes used to hide money or conceal a small weapon. Today the sash is often used to indicate the student's grade.

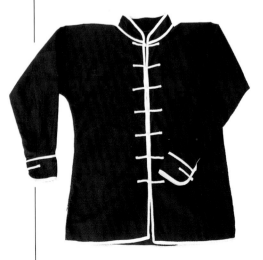

FOOTWEAR

Traditional shoes were often soft leather, or rope-soled 'slipper' types that were tied to the feet or lower leg by means of thin cord or rope.

In most modern Tai Chi schools students wear traditional Chinese-style cotton 'slippers', but many students train in modern trainers (sports shoes).

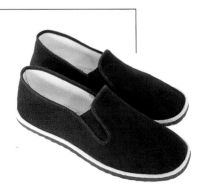

WEAPONS

When students have reached a required level of proficiency (which differs from school to school), a weapon of some sort is introduced into the training. Weapons are an intricate part of martial arts training and add an important dimension to it.

There is a certain etiquette to the use of weapons and different perspectives to consider. The weapon is not regarded as separate from the body, but as an extension of it. It is not an object to be waved around in any old manner, or played with casually.

Weapon forms, and the type of weapons offered, differ from school to school. Two weapons are usually used, the Straight Sword *(Chien)* and the Broadsword *(Dao)*, although not all schools offer both options. Some also offer a third weapon, the Staff, a wooden pole roughly 1.8m (6ft) long.

Starting weapons instruction is determined by the length of time the individual has spent training in his or her respective school. Students who show dedication and promise may be invited to participate in weapon training sooner than others.

Weapon etiquette is also taught. This normally consists of how to carry the weapon correctly, how to hold the weapon, greeting seniors when you have a weapon in your hand, greeting the weapon prior to touching it and after returning it to its resting place.

The swords used in Tai Chi are depicted below. Figures 1 and 2 show two wooden swords, which are generally used for practice if metal swords are not available. Figure 3 shows the sword and scabbard (holder) of the *Chien.* Figure 4 shows the *Dao.*

When using swords, the practitioners' energy becomes endowed within the sword, so it is preferable to have one's own sword rather than share another practitioner's weapon.

The material used to make swords is traditionally found in nature: wood is grown, and metal is extracted from the earth. Aluminium is regarded as a 'dead' metal, lacking in vital energy.

GRADING

The need to measure progress has resulted in most Tai Chi schools offering some form of 'grading', normally in the form of an exercise routine incorporating the movements learned since the last grading. Some schools have rather elaborate ceremonies accompanying the grading; others are more simple and straightforward.

Levels of grading differ from school to school, and uniforms often reflect the levels within each school.

Coloured shirts or sashes signify the various grades that can be attained. The shirts often have the school's emblem or badge on the front.

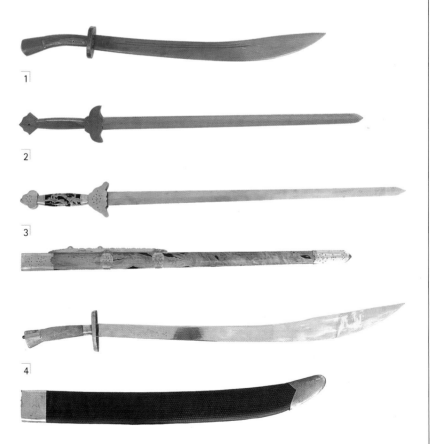

CONCEPT OF CHI

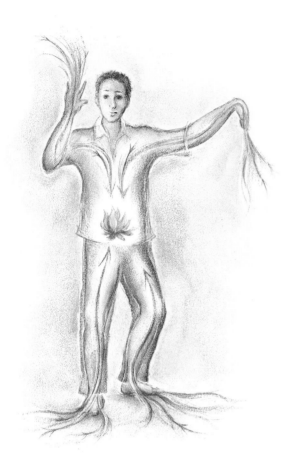

For centuries, the Chinese have studied the concept of chi. According to Chinese medicine, the body has pathways through which chi flows, providing energy and life. These pathways, or meridians, don't follow veins and arteries, but appear to have a close relationship with the lymphatic system, although there is nothing to substantiate this. The meridians cannot be seen, nor analyzed by an autopsy or by X-ray. They are not so much physical as metaphysical.

In Chinese medicine, many forms of sickness and ill health are considered to result from a blockage of chi, or an interruption in the free flow of chi through the body. Treatment consists of stimulating various points on the body by means of massage or acupuncture so that the free flow of chi is restored to the body and the individual's health improves. This concept of the flow of chi is carried into the martial arts, and is regarded as an integral part of the training.

Chi is cultivated and stored in the body by the regular practice of certain exercises. The area in which it is stored, known as the *Tan Tien*, is situated roughly three finger-widths below the navel. It is often illustrated as a small pot. Chi is closely linked to breath – as we breathe air in, so we breathe in chi. It is important to be able to visualize chi entering the body. This visualization can take the form of light, or a light mist, and aids one in the development of chi in the body. If one visualizes chi, it will exist.

There are many facets to the study of the different types of chi and its relationship to the body. The in-depth study of it is known as *Chi Kung* or *Qigong*.

In the 'hard' styles of Kung Fu, rigorous physical routines, known as Iron Body training, condition the body to 'become as iron' and therefore almost impervious to physical blows. These physical routines are often combined with exercises which cultivate the chi and enable the student to develop extremely powerful techniques.

'CONCEPT' is defined as 'an idea or general notion'. In the practice of Tai Chi Chuan, it is important to accept the notion of the existence of chi, and keep the idea of chi alive in the mind. A Chinese word, chi, or *qi,* does not translate well. The closest approximation is 'vital energy' or 'life force'.

Chi exists within us and without, it is the energy that binds all living things together. It is inherent in the body, it is not mystical or magical, and we all carry it with us. Certain exercises or activities increase the level of chi in the body, and with this we reduce the possibility of ill health.

Iron Body training focuses on the projection of chi from the body so that when contact is made, the chi is projected from the hand or foot directly into the target area. The objective of this is twofold; firstly, there is the shock and power of the actual blow; and secondly, the projection of chi into the target area is aimed at disrupting or damaging the internal organs. The idea of projecting chi is very important from a martial arts' sense, and is generally found throughout the Martial Arts of China.

In the 'soft' styles, these rigorous physical routines have tended to be replaced by others of equal importance. The exercises for the cultivation of chi also differ in the soft styles, and their focus alters somewhat.

As chi is linked to breath, so breath is linked to movement. By adjusting breath to match movement, we can generate chi. This is a very basic idea behind the practice of Tai Chi Chuan.

Movements are practised at a pace that increases the heart rate and gets the blood flowing faster through the body and limbs, while ensuring that breathing is comfortably controlled, so that the practitioner is able to breathe deeply and naturally throughout an entire set of movements.

Left **Chi is stored in the Tan Tien; the free flow of chi is central to understanding the movements of Tai Chi.**

As the practitioner moves through the postures, the act of breathing in and out becomes matched to certain movements. Breathing out is normally associated with movements that extend outward from the body, while breathing in is associated with movements drawing towards the body. An increase in the heart rate increases the blood flow. When this is combined with deep regular breathing, the amount of oxygen supplied to the body is increased. Because chi is linked to breath, this translates into an increase in the amount of chi in the body.

As the practitioner becomes more adept at the movements of Tai Chi Chuan and the body gains strength, the stances become lower and more extended. The movements are such that muscles, ligaments and joints are kept in constant motion. As the blood flows faster through the veins and arteries, so the chi flows more quickly through the various meridians.

With the chi flowing, the chance of blockages in the meridians is reduced. Therefore the regular practice of Tai Chi Chuan increases the amount of chi flowing through the body and reduces the likelihood of illness.

When a Tai Chi student reaches what his or her teacher judges to be a sufficient level of knowledge, the exercise called 'Pushing Hands' will be introduced *(see page 80)*. This exercise is performed with a partner and is a

backward–forward movement routine with the partners' hands and wrists in constant contact. The aim of the exercise is to become aware of the shifting energies of chi within the body, in order to utilize one's chi in a more practical manner.

By becoming sensitive to an opponent's chi, the practitioner can judge what type of attack is to be launched in his or her direction. By sensing that an opponent is committed and cannot retract, the practitioner's own attack can be directed in a desired direction and a counterattack launched.

Chi is best developed and cultivated through slow rhythmic movements that are matched to a breathing pattern. The development of chi is linked to a healthier, stronger body and with regular practice, one soon feels the added benefits. Chi revitalizes the body, not just physically, but also mentally and spiritually. One is left feeling more alive, more aware, less fatigued and with more energy to enjoy life.

If you are interested in developing your chi, it is important to work with a teacher who specializes in Chi Kung. Chi energies are complementary to the study of Chinese Martial Arts, but if the development of chi is not properly guided, its effects can be reversed and may cause illness. If cultivated correctly, chi will allow you to lead a fuller, more active life, with added energy, vitality and health.

THERE are many aspects to learning Tai Chi Chuan, from breathing correctly to understanding how the body works. No matter how deeply involved you become, there never seems to be an end to what can be learned. Learning Tai Chi is not a quick process, but unlike many things in life – what you put into the art will come back tenfold.

Regard Tai Chi in the same way as you would consider an investment in your future. With proper planning and forethought, your money will grow so that you may retire in comfort someday. Likewise, the regular practice of Tai Chi Chuan in your early years will pay dividends in the form of improved health and wellbeing, enabling you to enjoy your retirement years with vigour and a spring in your step.

Readers should note that this book is not meant as a replacement tool for training. It is simply a guide to a better understanding of the subject, as there can be no substitute for learning from a qualified instructor.

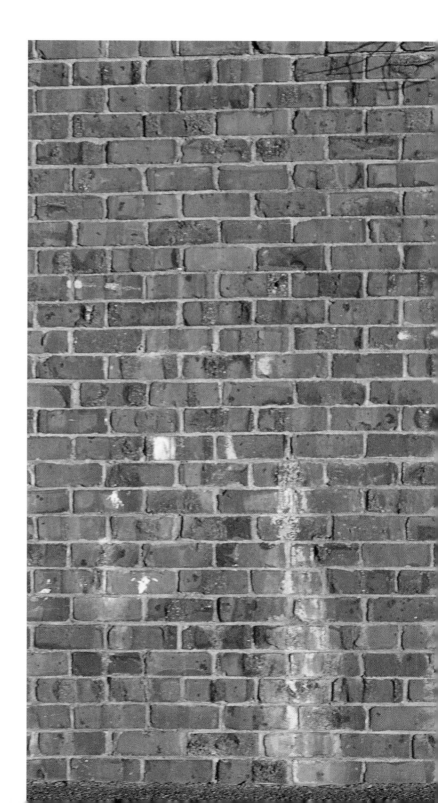

BEGINNING TAI CHI

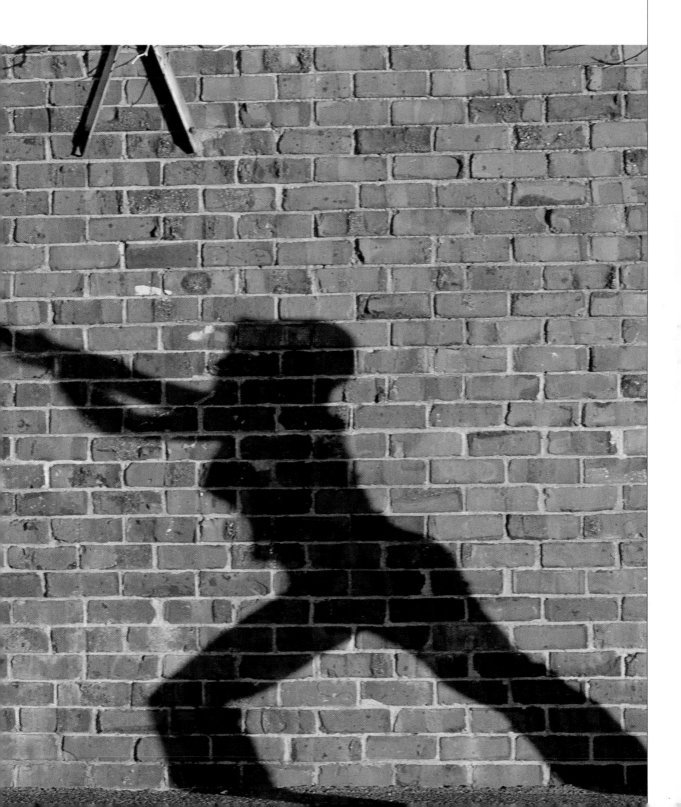

PREPARATION FOR PRACTICE

THE hardest part of any new activity is finding the time in a usually busy lifestyle to practise it. The first step to practising Tai Chi Chuan is to put time aside, either in the morning or evening, for oneself. It does not need to be a lot of time at first, but try to start off with about 30 minutes. Once you have begun a regular 30-minute routine, it will become easier to increase the allotted time. If it is possible, try to be outdoors. Otherwise choose a room that is not too cluttered, so that you have room to move freely. Ideally, it should also have ample natural light, and a free flow of air (try to avoid draughty or windy places). Find a place that offers a sense of tranquillity and calm.

It is important to try to establish a regular daily routine and build the habit of taking this time for yourself. You may wish to train only every second day in the beginning. That is fine, but try to take the same amount of time every day. On alternate days, you could work through breathing exercises, or use the time as a period to unwind at the end of the day or prepare yourself for the day ahead. Ultimately, the goal is regular daily practice.

When you begin practising Tai Chi Chuan, start off slowly and build up. As with many other things in life, developing a strong foundation in the movements is important and although sometimes your progress may seem slow, don't worry about it too much. Try not to complicate things – a movement or concept may initially look more difficult than it really is. The eye often tricks us into seeing complications that are not actually there. Don't force yourself to adapt to too many new ideas or concepts in the beginning, and don't analyze or intellectualize too much. Westerners have acquired the habit of analyzing. Sometimes the simple acceptance of an idea or concept is closer to the truth than the analysis of it.

Take the discovery of a new plant, as an example. In the West, scientists would dissect and examine every facet of the leaves, flowers and roots in order to better understand the plant's properties and characteristics, but they would have to kill the plant in order to do this. However, scientists working in Eastern traditions would study and observe the plant as a living organism, and so it would live.

The intrinsic difference between these two paradigms lies in learning how to accept what *is,* as this often gives a clearer picture than analyzing what *is not.*

The Tao teaches us that we are part of nature, and practising Tai Chi helps us to live in harmony with it.

Above **Take time to build a strong foundation. In the same way as a tree grows roots to anchor and nourish it, getting the basics right is the key to developing in Tai Chi Chuan.**

ATTITUDE

WHEN beginning Tai Chi, it is important to develop or cultivate an attitude of 'relaxed awareness'. The idea behind this is that you should be relaxed physically as well as mentally, yet remain aware of the body and its surroundings. True relaxation is not about 'letting go', rather, it is about being alert and entering a heightened state of receptivity and openness.

An awareness of one's surroundings is not a gift – it is a quality that can be developed and practised. Far too many of us have a tendency to pass through life with very little actual awareness of what surrounds us in our daily existence.

To help develop your own level of awareness, find a place, either indoors or outdoors, where you feel comfortable. Sit quietly and look around you at various objects in your vicinity. Look at their shape, size, colour and where they are in relation to where you are sitting. Take this all in, and then close your eyes and, sitting totally still, imagine that you are looking at those very objects. See them in your mind, and place them in their relationship to where you are.

Mentally try and judge the distance between yourself and each object, and their distance from each other. Then, still with your eyes closed, listen to the sounds around you, trying to place them in context; breathe deeply and smell the air to see if you can identify any scents or odours you may detect.

In other words, try and pick up a 'sense' of your surroundings. With regular practice, this will enhance your awareness of your surroundings.

As we become more aware of our surroundings, we become familiar with them, and as the feelings of familiarity increase, our levels of relaxation and awareness increase.

As our overall awareness increases, our awareness of ourselves grows, giving us a better understanding of how our bodies move, and of our relationship to the world around us.

Understanding these concepts is very important when we perform the movements of Tai Chi Chuan.

Cultivating the correct attitude for the practice of Tai Chi Chuan not only enhances our understanding of the movements, and the way we perform them, but carries over into our daily lives to offer us a renewed quality of life. Learning how to be relaxed, calm, and have a clear mind at all times is fundamental to the successful practice of Tai Chi.

Below **Developing an awareness of one's surroundings helps to cultivate the right attitude for Tai Chi.**

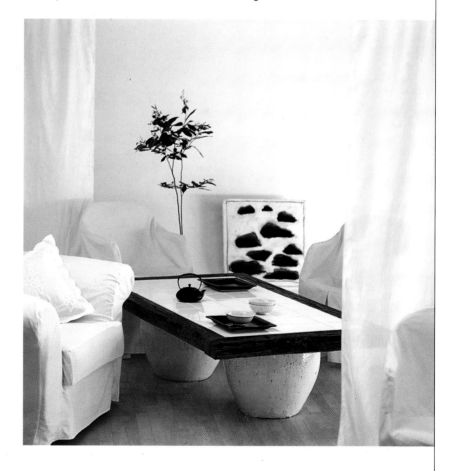

WARMING UP

WARMING UP before any form of exercise is important. It loosens the joints and muscles, strengthens them and allows free-ranging movements. It builds up the heart rate, relieves stiffness and enhances the flow of oxygen to the body. Warm-up exercises should be easy and uncomplicated and should not leave you tired. Although Tai Chi Chuan is generally performed at a slow tempo, warming up allows us to maintain the fluidity of movement necessary to attain the desired results.

In cold climates, warming up should take longer than in warm climates or during summer. Practising in the morning normally requires a longer warm-up period than in the afternoon or early evening.

Warming-up exercises may differ from school to school, or from teacher to teacher. Those presented here are a small sample of what is available.

FROG SIT (below)

This exercise strengthens the legs, tones and stretches the muscles, and loosens the joints from hips to ankles.

Place the feet shoulder width apart ensuring the feet are parallel to each other. Reach down and place both hands on the feet, while bending the legs into a squatting position (1) with the elbows on the inside of the knees, exerting a little pressure outwards. Keep the head up, as this ensures the spine is straight.

With the hands on the feet, slowly straighten the legs until they are fully extended (2), then return to frog sit.

When starting, try to hold the position for 30 seconds, then straighten the legs for 10–15 seconds. Once you are comfortable with that, continue to increase the squatting time until you reach two minutes. The amount of time for keeping the legs straight can remain at 15 seconds.

Points to remember:

• Make sure the posture is correct.
• Keep the head up.
• Make sure the elbows are on the inside of the knees.
• Don't allow the buttocks to drop too far. Try to keep the upper leg area, from behind the knee to under the buttocks, parallel to the floor.
• When straightening up, keep the movement slow and steady.

LEG EXTENSION (above right)

This exercise allows the muscles and ligaments of the inner leg to stretch and warm up prior to doing the splits.

From the frog sit position, keep the hands on the feet and shift the weight slowly onto the right leg while extending the left leg (1). Try to stay at the same level and keep the buttocks as low as possible. Slowly shift the weight back to the centre (2), and repeat the movement on the other side.

If a lack of flexibility won't allow you to keep a hand on your foot at all times, then hold the ankle as close to the foot as you can. Flexibility and suppleness will increase with practice.

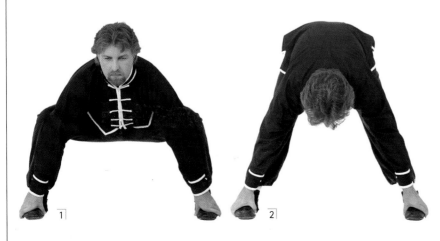

1

2

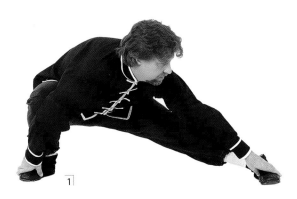

1

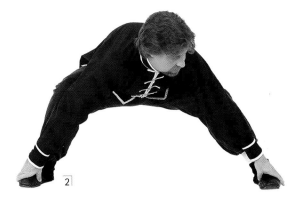

2

Points to remember:

- Stay as low as possible.
- The extended leg must be straight, with no bend at the knee.
- The knee of the bent (supporting) leg must be outside the elbow.
- Keep the buttocks down through the transition.
- Try not to bend the back too much. There will be some bending, but try to keep it to a minimum.
- Keep the transition at a steady pace and do not move too fast.

A variation is to reach the extension and, with the hand on the extended foot, revolve the foot on the heel so that the toes point upwards, then pull the toes towards you.

SPLITS (below)

Splits loosen and strengthen the leg muscles, allowing greater flexibility and a larger range of leg movement. From the leg extension (2 above), place both hands flat on the floor and slowly slide the legs outwards until they are fully extended on either side. Hold the posture for one minute. Revolve the feet on the heels and turn the toes up to face the ceiling. With the toes up, hold for one minute more.

Walk your hands backwards, supporting your weight, until you are sitting down with your legs spread out on either side (not shown). To end, place both hands on the outside of the knees and push the legs together. Bend the knees and bring the legs up to the chest. Place your arms around your legs and hug them to your chest to help relieve tension in the muscles. Once you are comfortable with a minute, increase each posture in 30-second increments. Aim for a hold of five minutes for each posture, but don't expect miracles to begin with.

Points to remember:

- Keep the soles of the feet **flat** on the floor.
- When turning the toes up, try not to shift too much weight backwards. Some shift will occur, but try to keep it to a minimum.
- Keep the wrists in line with the toes. This ensures that the body weight is over the hips. If the hands are too far forward, the arms carry the weight and pressure is exerted on the lower back.
- Control the sit down, don't just flop backwards.

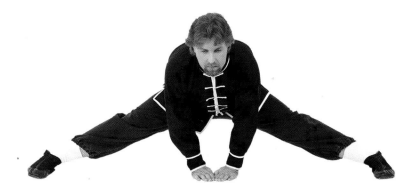

TWISTING TORSO (right)

This exercise loosens up the spine from the waist to the neck and helps to relax the muscles of the upper back, shoulders and neck.

To begin, the feet should be roughly shoulder width apart, turned slightly inward, with the knees slightly bent (1). This ensures that at the furthest point of the turn no unnecessary twist or pressure is placed on the opposite knee. Keep the arms hanging loose and shoulders relaxed.

Gently turn the body from side to side (2–5), allowing the arms to swing freely. Gradually speed up. The head must turn with the torso and the body should remain as relaxed as possible. Keep the spine erect and don't shift the weight from leg to leg as you turn. The idea is to twist the spine without leaning in any particular direction.

Start with two minutes, building up to five minutes. If you have a back or spine injury, consult your physician before attempting this exercise.

Points to remember:

• Keep the feet turned slightly inward and flat on the floor.

• Keep the legs slightly bent.

• Keep as upright as possible and don't shift the weight from leg to leg.

• Keep the arms and shoulders relaxed and loose.

• Turn the head and look behind you on each turn, keeping the head up in a natural position.

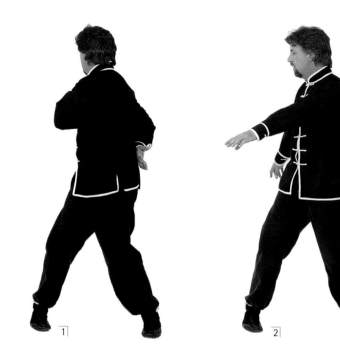

1

2

SWINGING ARMS (below)

This loosens up the shoulders and elbows. Keep the movements easy and keep the body upright yet relaxed. Don't tense the shoulders. Alternate left arm over right, right over left.

Begin by standing with the legs apart and feet parallel, toes forward.

Extend the arms (1) out to each side, until roughly shoulder height. Allow the arms to swing down and over one another (2).

Points to remember:

• Relax the shoulders and neck.

• Keep the body upright, but with a minimum amount of tension.

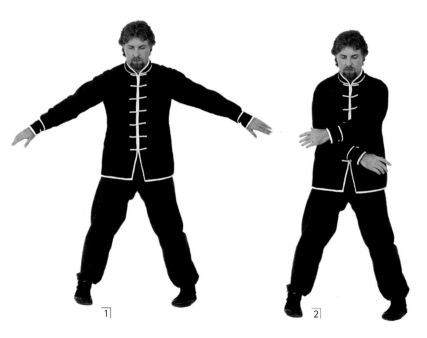

1

2

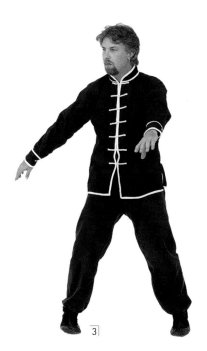

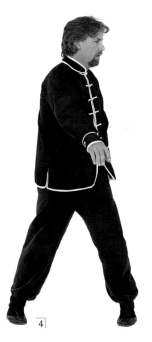

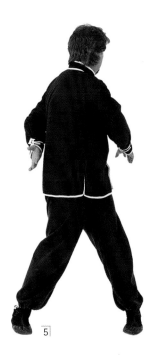

3   4   5

WRISTS (below)

This exercise loosens the wrists and warms up the muscles and tendons of the forearms. Interlock the fingers and bring the elbows towards each other in front of the body, so the forearms are almost touching. Slowly revolve the wrists with a forward rolling motion (1 – 4). Repeat with a backward rolling motion. Increase the speed until you are revolving the wrists vigorously. Between one and two minutes is sufficient. Points to remember:

- Relax the shoulders and arms.
- There should not be any undue movement of the arms as a whole.

STANDING PUSH UPS (not shown)

These strengthen the upper arms and shoulders. Stand facing a wall, more than an arm's length away. Raise your heels off the floor and, with your arms extended, lean towards the wall, supporting yourself in a classic 'push up' position and ensuring your back remains straight. Bend your arms to bring your nose closer to the wall, then push away again.

Variations include using only your fingertips to touch the wall. Begin with 15 repetitions per variation and go up in increments of five reps at a time. Make the exercises harder by moving your feet further away from the wall.

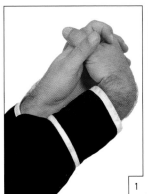

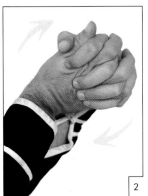

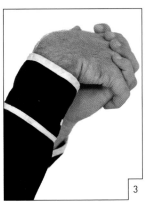

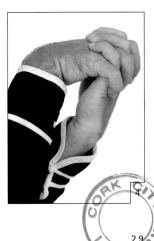

1   2   3   4

PREPARATION POSTURE

EVERYTHING has a starting point, and Tai Chi Chuan is no different. The physical starting point in this case is a body posture. Most of the Tai Chi Chuan forms start from this preparation posture, which is also termed grounding or centreing.

When we adopt the preparation posture, we ground the body to the earth through the legs and feet, and centre the body in a vertical position. We also centre the mind on what is to come, and centre the essence of life, or chi, in the *tan tien* area, which is located three finger widths below the navel *(see page 20)*.

Taking two or three deep abdominal breaths *(see page 32–33)* after settling

into the preparation posture helps to establish a strong, comfortable and relaxed stance before starting any other movements.

Throughout the forming of the preparation posture, the body should remain relaxed and as upright as possible, with the least amount of strain. The step out should be slow and controlled, but not too slow. From the start with the feet together, through to the final settlement in the centre, should take about seven seconds.

Begin by standing with the feet together, back as straight as possible, head upright and arms, shoulders and neck relaxed (1). Slowly bend the legs and take your weight onto the right leg

(2–3). Step out to the left with the left foot, keeping it just off the floor, and place the ball of the foot on the floor (4). Push the heel out slightly (5) and slowly shift the weight from the right leg back towards the centre (6).

Continue shifting the weight until it is on the left leg. Lift the ball of the right foot slightly, keeping the heel off the floor, and turn the foot slightly inwards (7). End by shifting the weight back to the centre (8).

When you are learning, check your feet while stepping out and settling, but as you familiarize yourself with the movements, keep your head up and look forward. Relax the shoulders and neck area as much as possible.

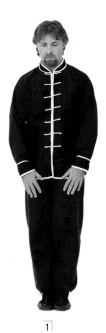

1

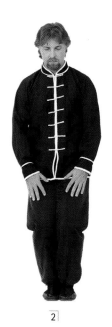

2

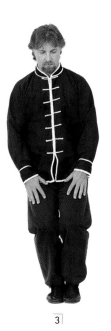

3

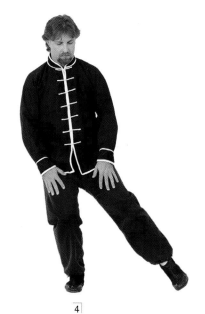

4

When the feet are placed correctly, they should be roughly shoulder width apart, with the outsides of the feet parallel to each other, and the knees slightly bent, so that the leg muscles help to absorb the body weight. (Play with the distance between your feet, moving a little either way until you find your most comfortable position.) Practise this sequence regularly, until it becomes a totally natural process.

The hands are neither to the side of the body, nor on the front of the leg. They lie in a natural position, roughly midway between the side and front. Find this by standing with your feet slightly apart and shrug (lift) your shoulders. Release the shrug and let your arms dangle freely. Make sure that the arms are in this position when practising the preparation posture.

Try breathing through the movement cycle. Breathe in as soon as you start bending the legs and continue the in-breath until you reach full capacity (as the ball of the left foot is being placed on the ground). Now breathe out through the rest of the movement until settling in the centre.

When one is centred, it is important that the spine is correctly aligned. When standing normally, the spine curves slightly inward just above the pelvic bone. This places strain on the lower back, which can be relieved by tilting the pelvis slightly forwards in an upward direction to bring the spine into alignment.

Points to remember:
• Keep the neck and shoulders relaxed.
• Tilt the pelvis to bring the spine into alignment.

• Allow the hands to lie naturally.
• Make sure the outsides of the feet are parallel.
• Ensure the legs are slightly bent.
• Don't over-emphasize the shifting of weight by leaning; stay upright.

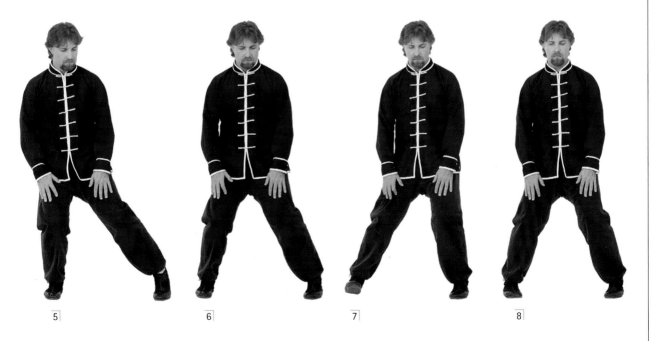

5   6   7   8

BREATHING

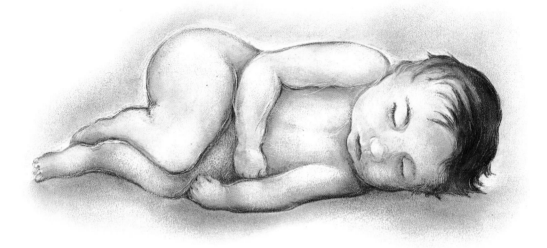

THE most important aspect in the practice of Tai Chi Chuan is learning to breathe correctly. Considering that the development of chi is linked to breath, incorrect breathing will prevent chi from being developed.

The method of breathing used in Tai Chi Chuan is termed abdominal breathing. This means that on breathing in, the stomach pushes outward, and on breathing out, the stomach retracts inward. This seems strange at first, but it is actually a very natural way of breathing.

Babies and young children automatically use abdominal breathing. It is only through growing up and going to school that we are taught to stand up straight, to pull the stomach in and push out the chest. While this may improve stance and posture, it is not conducive to breathing correctly. As adults, we have to relearn the proper process in order to obtain maximum benefit from our breathing.

When you begin using abdominal breathing, it may take concerted thought to practise it throughout the day. After a while though, it becomes less of a conscious thought and more of an instinctive action. Then a day will arrive when you are no longer aware of breathing in this manner, and your breathing pattern has become what it should naturally be.

Initially, it is normal to feel a little light-headed, because you are pulling more air into your body than it is used to. Your stomach muscles may also feel sore at first, because you are using them constantly. However, the increase in abdominal movement while breathing also aids the digestive system, and it is not unknown for bowel movements to increase in frequency or become more regular.

There are three basic methods by which we can take air in and expel it. Most schools of Tai Chi Chuan tend to use one breathing method in preference to the others.

The first method is to keep the jaw relaxed, with the lips slightly parted and breathe in and out through the mouth. This is easy and convenient, although the downfall is that, regardless of whether the air is either very cold or very hot, it is being pulled into the body in a direct manner. This hot or cold air then comes into contact with the bronchial tubes with little variation in temperature, so there is the possibility that bronchial problems may occur in some cases.

Above **Learning to breathe like a baby is the key to rediscovering how to obtain the maximum benefit from this essential life force.**

The second method is to keep the mouth closed while breathing in through the nose, and open it to breathe out (through the mouth). This is better from a point of view of hot or cold air intake, as the passage through the nose allows the air to either warm up or cool down to body temperature before reaching the bronchial tubes. The problem with this method is that each cycle of breath becomes a constant, conscious action of opening and closing the mouth.

The third method is to keep the mouth shut while breathing in and out through the nose. Although the mouth is closed, the jaw should remain relaxed. The tip of the tongue is often placed lightly on the roof of the mouth just behind the front teeth, to keep the flow of saliva alive in the mouth. The nose acts as a kind of filter, with the hairs of the nostrils filtering dust and other particles in the air.

The air has the opportunity to warm up or cool down to body temperature, as in the second method but, as there is no opening or closing of the mouth, the breathing cycle remains natural and thought-free. (Another benefit of this method is that if your mouth is shut, you can't put your foot in it!)

Right **Mastering abdominal breathing helps to maximize the free flow of chi energy into and through the body via pathways, or meridians.**

When you begin Tai Chi, start with the last technique described. It is not only the easiest method, but is also the one most commonly taught.

Practise abdominal breathing at every opportunity, so that it becomes your natural breathing pattern. The nice thing about this exercise is that it can be practised anywhere – in your car, on a plane, in the office, or in the comfort of your favourite chair.

The exercise is not only about breathing, the rhythmic action is also therapeutic in nature and assists relaxation. Change your breathing, change your life.

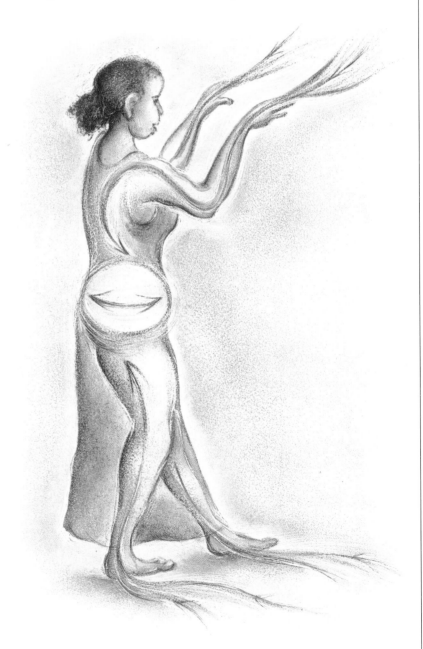

ROOTING

THE dictionary defines the word 'root' in many different ways, but the definition that applies here is 'the source or origin of a quality, the basis upon which anything rests, to fix or establish firmly'.

One of the lessons of life is that if the things we build do not have strong foundations, they are likely to fall over. Tai Chi Chuan is no different. If your basic postures are not strong enough, your ability to apply them will be hampered and your balance will be shaky and insecure.

When standing, the feet should be placed firmly on the ground. The weight of the body should be centred downward, and there should be a feeling of attachment to the ground. You should try and cultivate a sense of sinking or lowering of the energy of the body. Try to imagine the body's energy draining downward to settle in the legs and abdomen, below the waist and navel.

When you practise stepping *(see page 54)* pay close attention to the subtle changes of weight that occur throughout a step. As you place your

Right **The feet should have a feel of growing roots with every step – only you have the ability to move them from where you have placed them.**

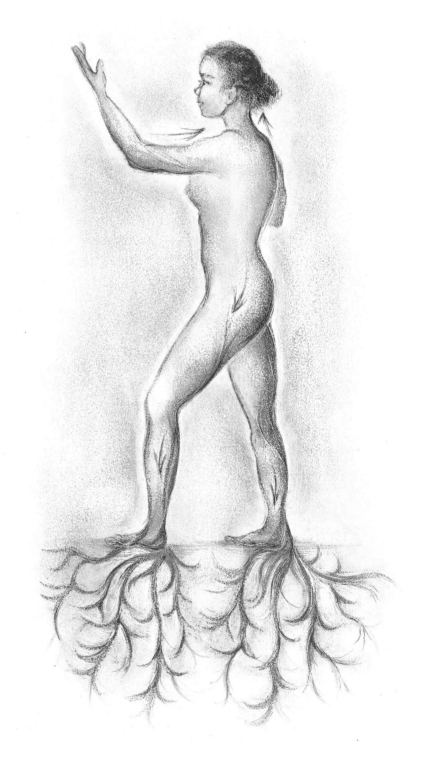

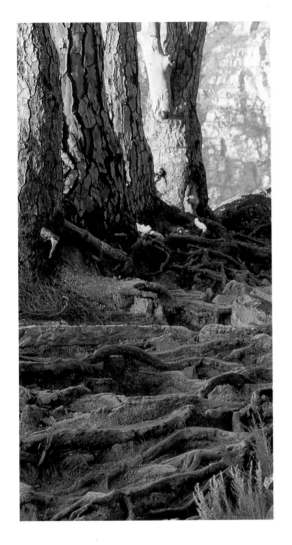

feet down there should be a sense of them taking root or growing roots. Once placed, they should be unable to be moved from their position, unless allowed by you. There should be a sense of solidness and heaviness to your stance, but it is important that this is not a physical heaviness – you are not making yourself heavier by lowering your stance.

Maintain a sense of balance. If you need to shift weight to one leg, do it smoothly and evenly and be sure of your centre of gravity before moving or shifting your weight. The concept of rooting should be considered throughout the move. If you have all your weight on one leg, that leg should be well 'rooted' to support the rest of your body.

Breathing correctly is important for developing the sense of rooting, and abdominal breathing assists this development. The breath flowing down towards the abdomen encourages the chi to follow. As the chi flows it settles. This settlement is, in essence, a lowering or rooting of the body's energy.

Keep the concept of rooting alive in your mind at all times and throughout all the movements. Tai Chi Chuan is not simply a set of physical movements – practitioners are often required to visualize abstract concepts, one of which is the idea of rooting. 'Where the mind goes, the chi follows' – visualize the concept and it will occur.

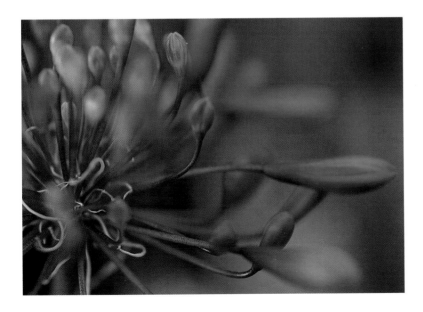

Top Rooting is an abstract concept that describes how energies are drawn downward in such a way as to bind us to the earth, the source of growth. Try to cultivate a sense of your energy sinking down towards the abdomen and from there into the legs.

Left Flowers only flourish when a plant has strong roots – and you will find that the way you practise Tai Chi will change with increased experience.

PRINCIPLES OF MOVEMENT

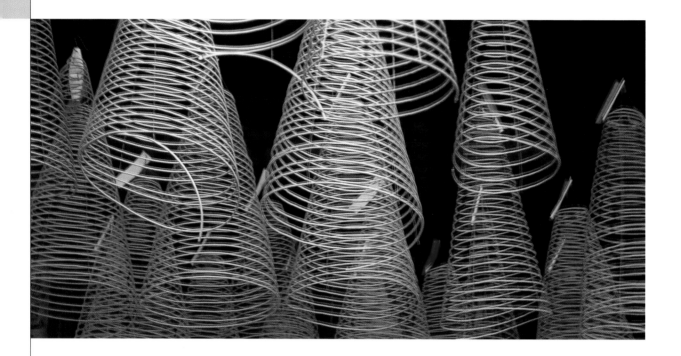

WHEN first attempting Tai Chi movements, try to maintain an even rhythm. It is important to remain relaxed throughout the exercises, yet be aware of the movements being performed and how the limbs are placed in relation to the rest of the body.

There will always be a certain amount of tension in one's body, but it should be the minimum necessary to hold or maintain the postures, with no dynamic tension or unnecessary stress placed on the muscles.

Physical movement should never be forced and it is important to keep all your movements as natural as possible. Your mind should be focused on each movement, or maybe one step ahead. Try not to let your thoughts wander too much, as this can result in movements becoming erratic and jerky. Try to settle your mind into a state of calm, quiet concentration. This state is almost meditative in nature, yet you are fully awake, aware of your surroundings, and focused on the movements at hand. In other words, attempt to mentally submerge yourself into the natural ebb and flow of the movements.

Coordination, which allows you to perform the exercises in a flowing manner, comes with regular practice and is not impossible to achieve.

Learning to coordinate movements to breathing is the first step, after which coordinating individual movements to one another becomes easier.

At first it is natural to feel that the limbs are totally out of sync with each other. This is generally due to the

Above **These spiral incense cones echo the flowing circles and curves that are the natural shapes promoted by Tai Chi Chuan exercises.**

Right **Coordination between hands and legs only comes with practise, but it is the key to developing grace and balance in all your movements.**

fact that almost all the sports and activities we participate in while growing up are geared towards speed, strength and endurance. Our minds are conditioned to think along those lines; they are not used to moving the limbs or body in slow motion. Training the body to move slowly starts in the mind and expresses itself outwardly into the physical movements.

Where other martial arts have a tendency to work along straight, direct lines, Tai Chi Chuan works in circles and curves. If one looks at the arms in their various postures, one sees that they curve slightly. Looking closer, one can see that this curve is actually following the line of least resistance on the limb. There is no undue bend on elbows or wrists, and when lifting or lowering the arms, the movements originate from the shoulders in a very natural way.

When watching Tai Chi Chuan for the first time, there is a tendency to think of it as being complicated and hard to perform. This is an illusion, caused by the manner in which the movements are strung together. The individual movements are, in fact, very simple and uncomplicated if one breaks them down to moving one limb at a time. It is the way in which the body moves as a whole that gives the illusion of being complicated.

When you begin, if you think of Tai Chi Chuan as being difficult, it will be, whereas if you focus on the simplicity and economy of the movements, it will become much easier. There are certainly subtleties and intricacies to the movements, but to start with, keep things simple. The other qualities can be acquired as you advance.

Tai Chi often appears to be an endless flow of movement. When starting out, it is normal to pause between postures to enable you to check that your body is correctly positioned. This is referred to as 'honouring the posture'. As you become familiar with the postures, the pauses between them will gradually become shorter, until the pauses become almost indiscernible and anyone watching will have the illusion that you are moving in a continuous flow.

Most importantly, relax. Tai Chi Chuan becomes easier to learn when the body is relaxed. At first this is hard, because there seems to be so much to consider. But as you continue to practise and familiarize yourself with the basic movements, the body will start to relax naturally. Once the physical relaxation starts to flow over onto your mental state, you will begin to find total relaxation in the practice of Tai Chi Chuan.

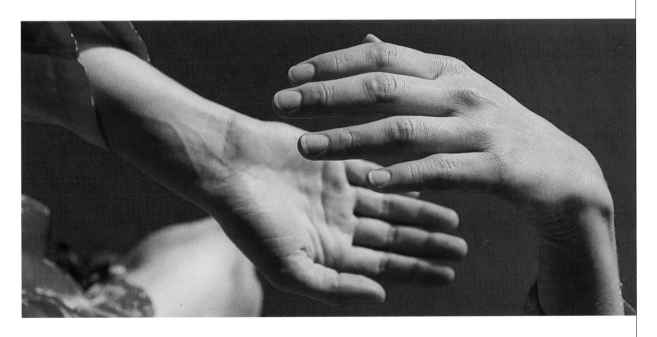

TAI CHI CHUAN *is a very powerful means by which to maintain a balanced lifestyle. It requires no special equipment; can be practised indoors or out; alone, with a partner for advanced exercises, or in classes, to enable you to become proficient-enough to practise the forms comfortably on your own.*

In motion the whole body should be light and agile, with all parts of the body linked as if threaded together like a string of pearls.
The ch'i (vital life energy) should be excited, the shen (spirit of vitality) should be internally gathered.
The postures should be without defect, without hollows or projections from the proper alignment; in motion, the Form should not become disconnected.
The chin (intrinsic strength) should be rooted in the feet, generated from the legs, controlled by the waist, and mani-fested through the fingers.
T'ai Chi Chu'an Ching
Chang San-Feng (c1279–1386)

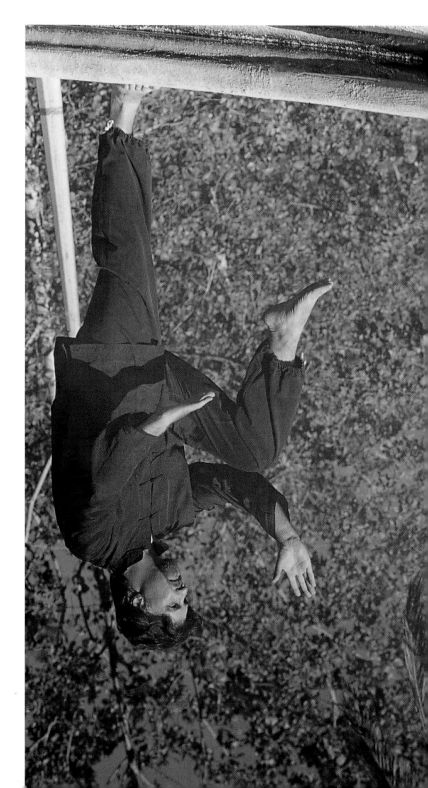

PRACTISING

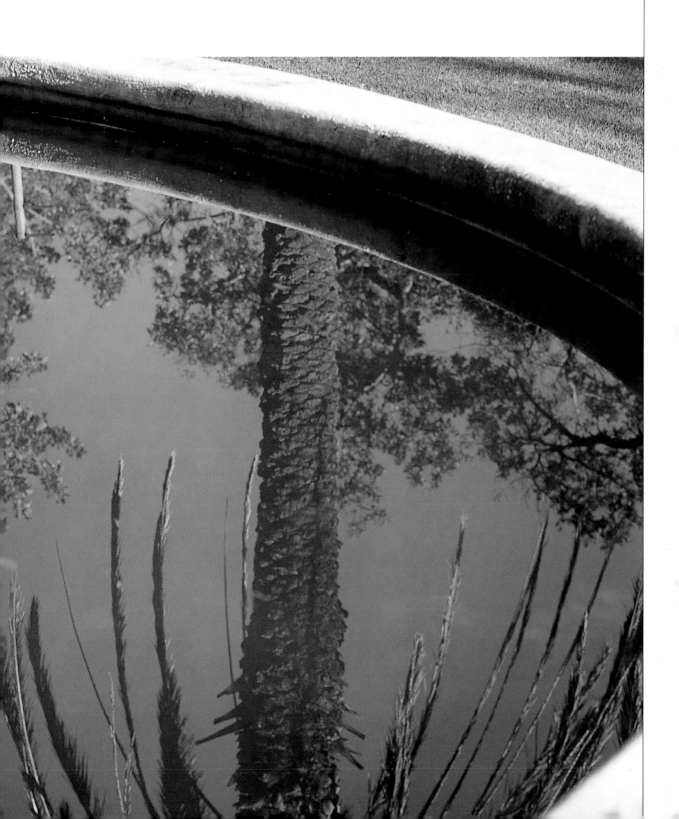

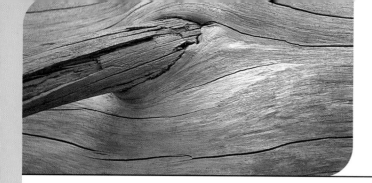

STANDING EXERCISES

THIS very basic exercise is light and easy, and can be done as a stand alone exercise. If you are practising a regular Tai Chi routine, do this after warming up, before beginning any of the actual movements, in order to slow the breathing, settle the heart rate, and focus on what is to come.

After a session, it is great as a means of winding down and relaxing, thinking of what you have done or learned.

Assume the preparation posture (1), lift the hands up in front of the body (2), palms facing one another. Now circle the arms as if you are trying to hug a tree (3). Make sure the fingertips are about 10cm (4in) apart and that the elbows don't point out to the sides, but droop slightly (4). The wrists should have a feeling of being suspended. The palms should face the body at about upper chest height.

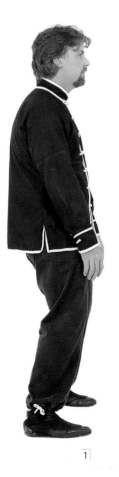

1

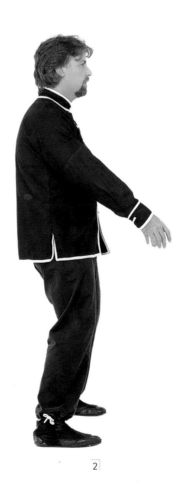

2

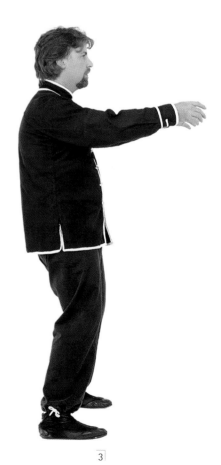

3

TRUNK CLASPING

Relax the shoulders and neck area. Close your eyes if you wish, and breathe deeply and naturally (5). Hold the posture for about three minutes to start with, and build up to eight minutes. Keep relaxed. There will be some muscle discomfort at first, but maintain the posture. If the arms begin to feel tired, lift them higher and push them out a little further; don't lower the arms until the time is up.

When you have finished the exercise, bend at the waist and allow the arms to hang downward. This relieves the tension in the shoulders.

To straighten up, bend the knees first, curve the back and slowly straighten up. Don't stand up with either the legs or the back straight.

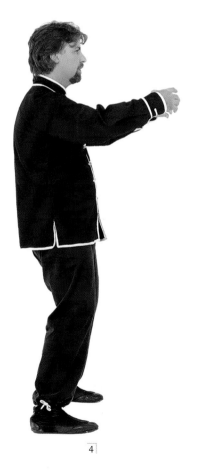

4

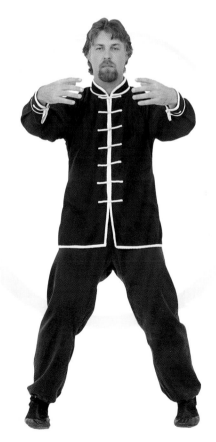

Front View

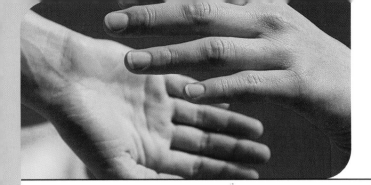

STANDING EXERCISES

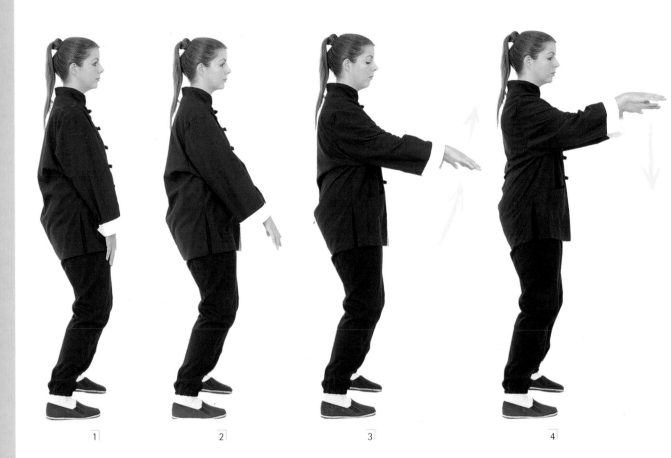

1   2   3   4

THIS exercise is taken from the opening posture of the 24-step form, also referred to as the Peking, or short, form.

Assume the preparation posture or stance (1) and relax for a moment. Lift the hands away from the body (2), wrists leading to shoulder level (3–4), then lower the hands, palm down (5–6), until they are in line with the hips (7). While lowering the hands, sink slightly lower on the legs.

It sounds too simple, so let's look at the movement more closely. Stand facing a wall or, preferably, a full length mirror or window. Assume the preparation stance and stand close enough to the wall, mirror or window so that, with your arms extended at shoulder height, you can place both hands flat on the surface. Then lower your hands to your sides.

Now move your hands away from your sides, towards the surface in front of you. As your fingertips come into contact with the surface, slide them gently over that surface as you raise your arms. The wrists will lead with the fingers trailing.

When the wrists reach shoulder height, change direction and move your fingertips back down the surface until you feel they are about to break surface contact.

RAISING & LOWERING
OF HANDS

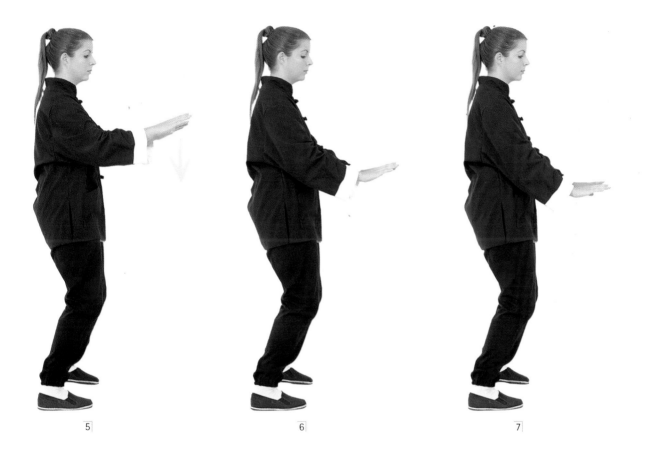

5 6 7

Stop moving the hands at this point. This will give you an indication of how far the hands should move away from the body before beginning to lift, and of where they should stop moving. Throughout this exercise, the shoulders and elbows should remain relaxed. The arms should not be turned or twisted in any direction.

Once you are comfortable with the feel of the raising and lowering movements, move away from the wall or window and try the movement in free space. Remember to sink slightly at the knees on lowering the hands.

To add a different quality to the movement, try abdominal breathing through the movement. Breathe in as soon as you start to move the hands, and continue the in breath until the wrists reach shoulder level. Breathe out from this point until the hands stop moving downward. Relax the hands back to their original starting position next to the legs and repeat the movement.

Practise this exercise until you are comfortable with both the movements and the breathing and they become totally in sync with one another.

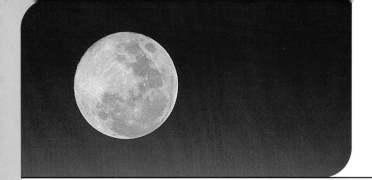

STANDING EXERCISES

THIS exercise introduces us to the concept of change and motion in a circular pattern, using an imaginary ball. All movement flows from the ball and returns to the ball.

Stand in the preparation posture and raise the arms out in front of you. Keep the hands roughly shoulder width apart and don't lock the elbows; relax them and the shoulders. The palms of the hands face each other in a relaxed state, there should be no tension in the hands or fingers. Lower the arms and allow the elbows to drift in slightly towards the body. Stop when they are roughly in line with the lower rib cage (1).

Move your hands so that you are supporting a ball between them and want to keep it there. Lower the right hand and raise the left hand (2–3) until the right hand would be directly under the ball, supporting it, and the left hand would be lying gently on the top of the ball (4).

Make sure the left elbow is relaxed slightly downward, not pointed to the side. Try this: with the left hand upper in the ball position, point the elbow to the side. Now drop the elbow slightly. The downward movement of the elbow is roughly 5cm (2in), but the tension is released altogether.

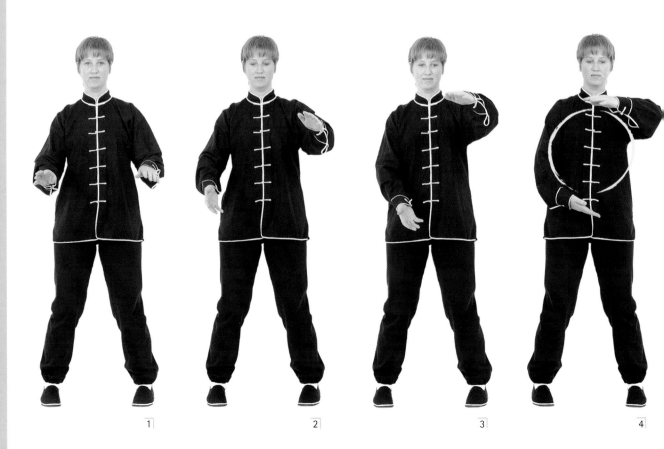

1   2   3   4

TAI CHI BALL

Throughout the movement, keep the arms and shoulders relaxed. Remember that it is important to maintain the least amount of muscular effort while moving the arms.

With the arms in the ball-holding position (4), pull them back towards the body and check the distance between the hands. The left hand should be in line with the underside of the chin and the right hand just below the navel.

Start the sequence again by rotating the hands into the ball (once again the left hand is over the right hand, as in 4). Now change the direction and move the right hand over the left hand (5–8). Keep rotating the ball slowly and gently, ensuring that the arms and shoulders are completely relaxed.

When you are comfortable with the movement, add the abdominal breathing. With one hand up and the other hand down, breathe in until the hands are halfway through the movement (shoulder width apart), then breathe out for the rest of the movement. Match the movements and breathing until the breathing almost dictates the movement.

Practise until the exercise becomes totally natural and comfortable before moving on to any of the other exercises.

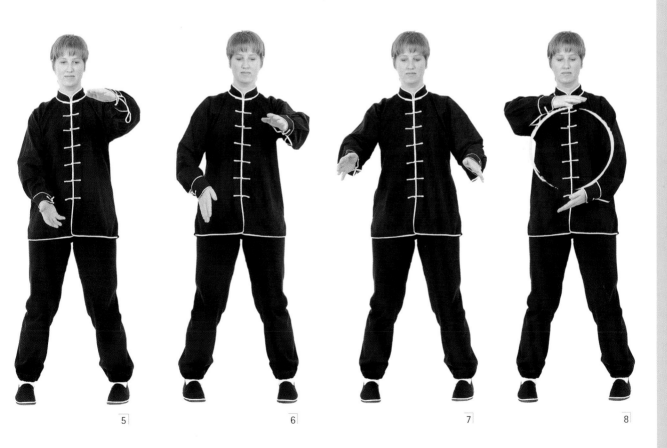

5   6   7   8

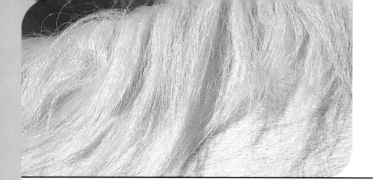

STANDING EXERCISES

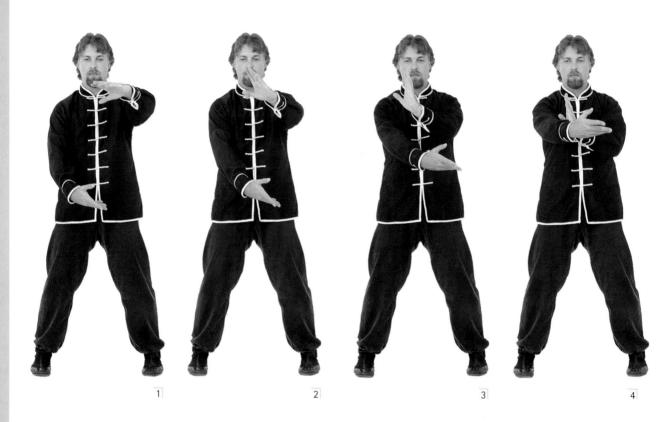

1	2	3	4

THIS is one of many movements that flow from the Tai Chi Ball. It allows us to develop a comfortable, natural extension to our movements, but requires some co-ordination.

Begin by assuming the preparation stance and form the ball with the left hand on top (1). Working with both hands, as depicted in the photographs, move the right hand across the body towards the left, and extend the hand upwards and outwards in a circular manner to stop in front of the right shoulder. Move the left hand across the body to just before the right shoulder, turning the hand vertically, then drop the left hand down and across the body to stop just in front of, and to the outside of, the left hip, with the fingers pointing forward and slightly inward (2–6). Ensure that the left hand drops down on the inside of the right arm, as shown in

picture 3, and crosses the inner elbow, as shown in picture 4 and that the right hand remains outside the left arm.

To learn this movement, it may be easier to first look at the quality of movement of each arm on its own. Begin by looking at the right arm only: The arm movement stems from the shoulder, and the elbow extends outwards only slightly through the movement. When the right hand is in front of the shoulder, the elbow points towards the floor and the wrist is relaxed. The fingers are not pointing straight out, but have a slight inwards curl due to the wrist being relaxed. The palm is also tilted slightly inward, allowing you to see the profile of the forefinger to the wrist uninterrupted by the thumb, as shown in picture 6, which shows the final position of the exercise.

PARTING
WILD HORSE'S MANE

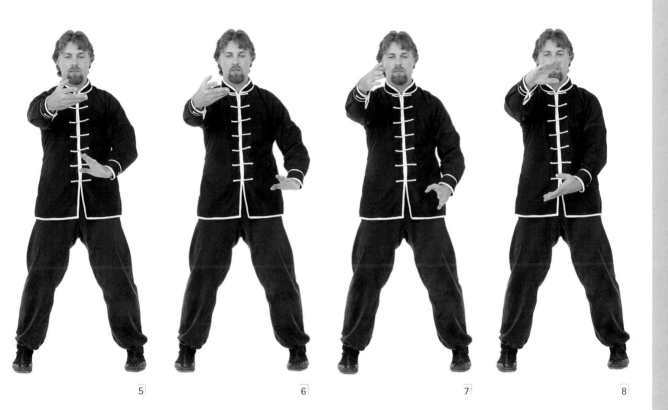

| 5 | 6 | 7 | 8 |

Now look at the left arm only: When you move the left hand across the body and turn it vertically, try to keep the fingertips on the same level. The wrist drops, the fingers don't lift. From its starting point, keep the hand the same distance from the body, don't allow it to drift in towards the body. It may draw in slightly when it stops, but no more than a hand-width away from the hip. In the left hand's final position, as shown in picture 6, the line of the wrist should be just in front of the body, with the elbow pointing in a backward direction. As before, the arm movement stems from the shoulder and the elbow remains relaxed throughout.

From the ball position, both hands should move and finish simultaneously. Neither hand must finish before the other. Once you have completed the movement, bring your forward hand back to form the upper hand of the ball, and the lower hand the base (7 and 8). This brings you back to the starting position (1), ready to repeat the exercise on the opposite side. As you work through the exercise, try to build up a flow from the Tai Chi ball into Parting Wild Horse's Mane and back into the ball in a repeating cycle. Keep your movements slow and steady, and pause at each full posture for a split second before moving on to the next.

Finally, add abdominal breathing. Breathe in while forming the ball, out through Parting Wild Horse's Mane, in as you reform the ball and out into the final posture.

Repeat this exercise until you feel totally at ease with the complete sequence, keeping the breathing slow to match each movement to your breath.

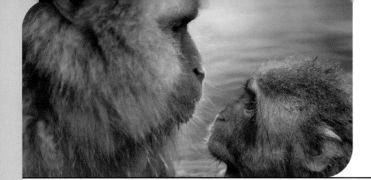

STANDING EXERCISES

THIS standing exercise adds the element of using the arms in conjunction with upper body movement, and introduces the idea of directing one's energy.

The exercise starts from the Tai Chi ball position, but from there the movements flow into one another, omitting the forming of the ball in-between.

Assume the preparation stance and form the Tai Chi ball in front of you, with your left hand uppermost (1). Drop the right hand down past the outside of the upper leg, and back up to shoulder level, simultaneously turning the upper body to face right. The right palm should remain up through the movement, and the eyes should follow the right hand with no undue movement of the head or twist of the neck.

At the same time, move the left hand forwards and upwards to shoulder level, as you turn the torso to the right, turning the left hand palm face up, with the arm just short of full extension (2-3). Remember that the head will follow the movement of the torso to the right.

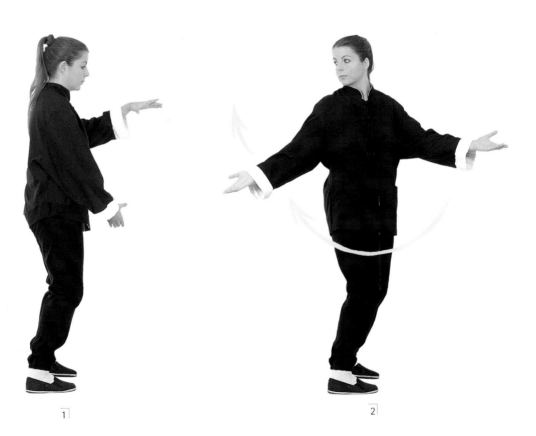

1

2

REPULSE MONKEY

Curl the right wrist so the fingertips face forward, and allow the right hand to drift forward as you start turning the torso back to face forwards. The right hand should drift past the head (as shown in 4), close to the ear, settling in front of the shoulder, with the arm just short of full extension and the elbow relaxed (5). Remember to use the minimum amount of strength in the arm to achieve the movement.

Simultaneously, allow the left elbow to bend and drop back towards the side of the body (4), stopping when it is next to the ribs, and forming a 90 degree angle, no more no less. In its final position; the left palm faces up, the left arm is as relaxed as possible, and the fingers face forward.

When the torso is facing right, the arms should be 180 degrees to one another at their furthest points (as shown in picture 3). As you curl the wrist of the back hand, simultaneously begin to turn the torso to face forwards while moving both hands towards their final resting places (6). The torso should finish moving as both hands settle into place.

continued on next page

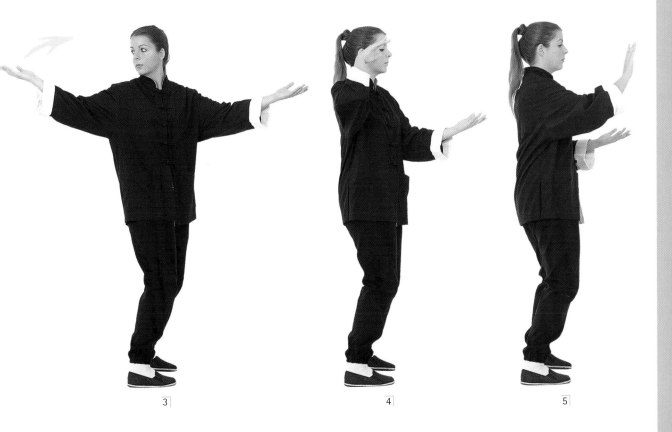

3   4   5

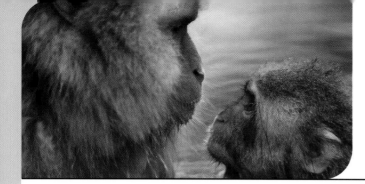

STANDING EXERCISES

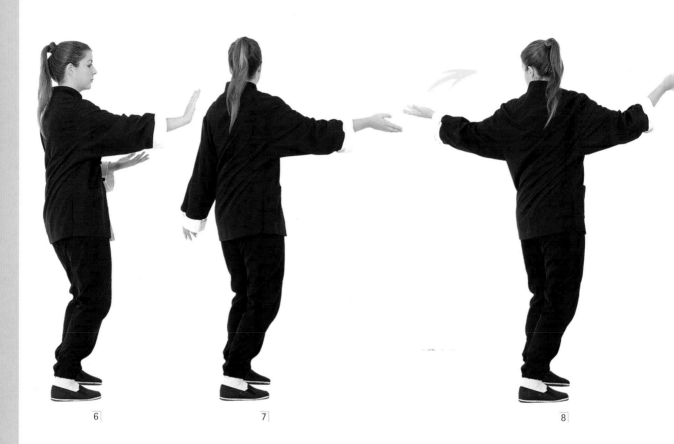

6

7

8

continued from previous page

This takes a little timing at first, but practise and play with the movement until you are comfortable and at ease with it.

If you started with the left hand upper on the Tai Chi ball, your right hand will be forward and the left hand down at your side (as shown in 6). Instead of reforming the ball, move the hands from where they are as you turn the torso to the left, to repeat the exercise on the opposite side (7–11).

In its final position, the forward hand must be in front of the shoulder. When this movement is used practically, as an application, the forward hand either absorbs energy coming into the body or projects energy into your opponent.

The following exercise should help to make this concept a little clearer. Stand in front of an open door and place your right hand on one side of the door, above the lock. Keep the fingers vertical and the arm slightly bent so that the elbow points towards the floor. Position your body so that your hand is in front of your shoulder. Gently lean towards the door, absorbing the weight on your arm by allowing the arm

REPULSE MONKEY

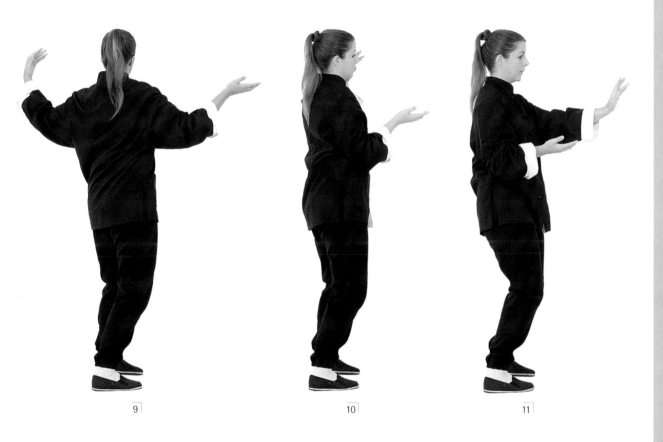

9   10   11

to bend. You should be able to support yourself quite comfortably on your arm. Now stand normally and reposition your body with the right hand in front of the left shoulder. Once again gently lean in towards the door, absorbing your weight by bending your arm slightly. Notice what happens.

Next, try positioning your body so your right hand is outside the right shoulder, and repeat the action. Both times the right hand will drift to the side, throwing you off balance. If the right hand is not positioned correctly, the energy of the body is misdirected, and this will throw you off balance or make you vulnerable. Always keep this in mind.

Once you are comfortable with the basic movements of Repulse Monkey, you can incorporate abdominal breathing in conjunction with the arm movements. Begin by breathing in as you turn and extend the arms, and breathe out as you settle into the final position.

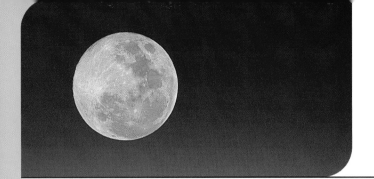

STANDING EXERCISES

THIS exercise develops the idea of shifting weight from one leg to another and helps to improve balance.

Assume the preparation posture, but don't worry about the hands for the moment; focus on the legs. Turn the left foot inward to roughly 45 degrees, and the right foot outward to roughly 45 degrees, absorbing the body's weight on the left leg (2). Do not lean in any particular direction, just shift the weight by moving the entire torso, hips to shoulders, as one. Hold the body upright. Lift the right knee upwards and back towards the chest (3–4). When you feel you have brought the knee up as far as is comfortable, swing the lower right leg forwards and extend it outward, keeping the toes pulled back and pushing forwards with the heel (5). When the leg is fully extended, hold for a split second, then pull the knee towards the chest, lower the leg and place the foot on the floor in the same position as before (6–8).

Throughout the leg extension, keep the body upright and supported by the left leg and do not lean backwards on the extension. When you begin, don't worry about leg height. It is important that you are able to fully extend the leg while maintaining the correct body posture. With practice your legs will strengthen and the height of the leg will increase.

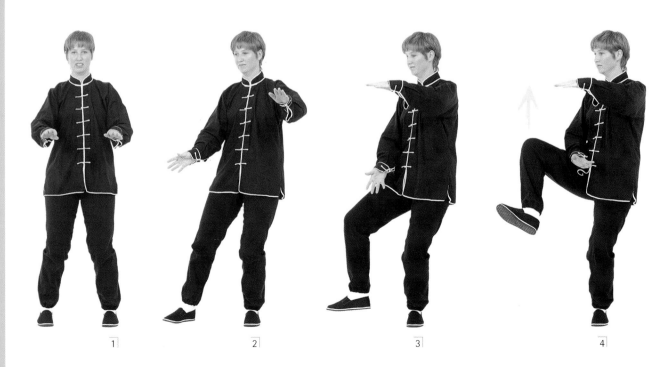

1   2   3   4

KICKING
WITH TAI CHI BALL

Once you have placed the right foot back on the floor, turn it inward to roughly 45 degrees and turn the left foot outward to 45 degrees, transferring the weight slowly throughout the entire process onto the right leg. Repeat the exercise on the left leg.

Keep alternating left and right legs until you are comfortable and familiar with the movements on both sides.

Now add the Tai Chi ball and the arm movements. Assume the preparation posture and turn the feet to the right while forming a ball with the left hand uppermost (1–3). Hold the ball throughout the kick and until the foot is placed back on the floor (4–7). Then, as you turn your feet and transfer the weight from leg to leg, change the ball. The ball should only stop moving as you are about to lift the foot off the floor. Keep playing with the ball as you alternate from leg to leg.

Once you are familiar with the physical movements of Kicking with Tai Chi Ball, add the abdominal breathing. Breathe in to start, and out through the first turn. Breathe in as you lift the leg, and out to the full extension; in on the withdrawal and foot placement, out through the turn; in with the lift in the other side; and so on. Remember to match each movement to a breath.

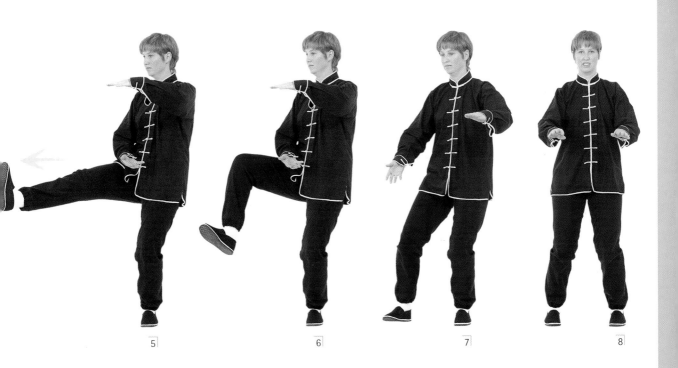

5 6 7 8

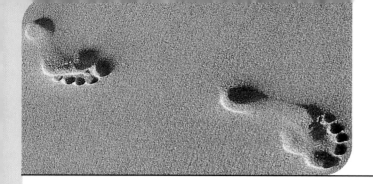

STEPPING - BASIC MOVE

STEPPING *adds movement to the lower half of the body and starts to bring the whole body into play. Practise stepping every day, as the quicker one becomes familiar with it the better.*

Start by standing with the feet about 7cm (3in) apart, both feet pointed straight forward. Turn the right foot out 45 degrees and, supporting your weight comfortably, bend both legs as far as you can. Begin by checking the placement of the foot: transfer the weight to the right leg, and move the left foot directly forwards, just off the floor. When the knee is straight, place the heel of the foot on the floor, with the toes pulled back toward you. Don't place any weight on the left foot yet. Check the placement of the foot, then draw the foot straight back and ensure that the gap is still apparent between the heels. This is very important; there must be a gap between the feet. If they touch when you bring the foot back, your stance will be too narrow and your balance will be poor.

To start the movement, bend the knees and take the weight on the right leg (1). Place the left foot forward with the toes pulled back and the heel touching the floor (2).

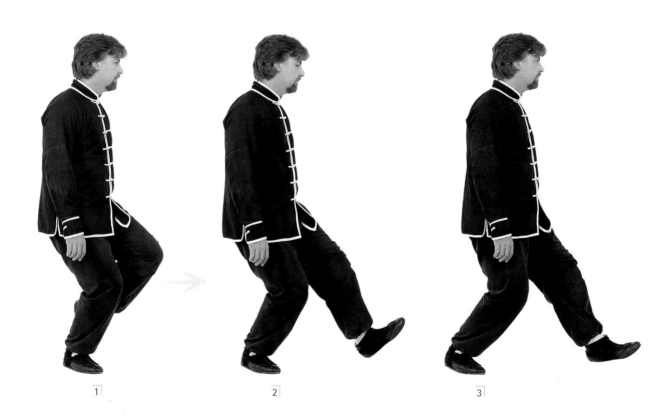

1

2

3

FORWARD STANCE

In this position the torso, from hips to shoulders, faces directly forward. Slowly transfer your weight onto the left foot as you flatten the foot (3). The hips move the torso forwards as you transfer your weight, and the torso remains comfortably erect throughout. Straighten the right leg as the weight transfers onto it and bend the left knee, keeping it pointed forward.

Look down and ensure that the tip of the foot protrudes slightly in front of the knee. If your knee covers your foot, you have gone too far, so adjust the stance accordingly.

The left foot must point directly forward, the heel of the right foot must remain on the floor, and the right leg must be straight; don't allow the knee to bend. Check your position and get a feel for the weight distribution on the legs. The torso should be erect and relaxed, with the arms hanging comfortably at the sides (4).

This position is known as a forward stance, and is where we begin stepping exercises from. Play with it until you are comfortable, then try the other stepping movements.

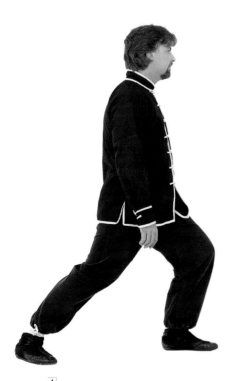

4

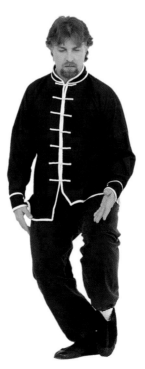

Front View 1

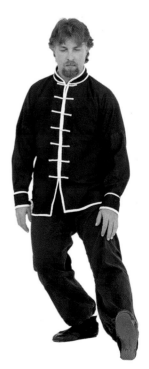

Front View 2

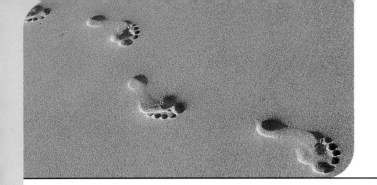

STEPPING - FORWARDS

ASSUME a forward stance, right foot forward (1). Shift the weight straight back onto the left leg, bending the knee to absorb the weight (2), and lift the toes of the right foot off the floor, pulling them back towards you (3). The right heel remains in contact with the floor. Swivel the right foot about 45 degrees to the right (4). Begin to transfer all the weight onto the right leg as you flatten the foot and bend the knee to absorb the weight. Keep the torso facing forward.

Once you feel comfortably balanced on the right leg, lift the left foot off the floor (5). Keep the knee of the left leg

pointed forward, and bring the left foot up past the middle of the calf muscle, practically brushing it with the outside of the big toe. Place the left foot on the floor, with the heel touching and the foot facing directly forward (6). Slowly transfer the weight onto the left leg as you flatten the foot (7) and assume a left forward stance (8). The step through to placing the heel down should be a smooth and uninterrupted motion. Gently place the heel on the floor; do not fall onto it. The knee must point forward at all times through the step forwards. Do not let it point out to the side.

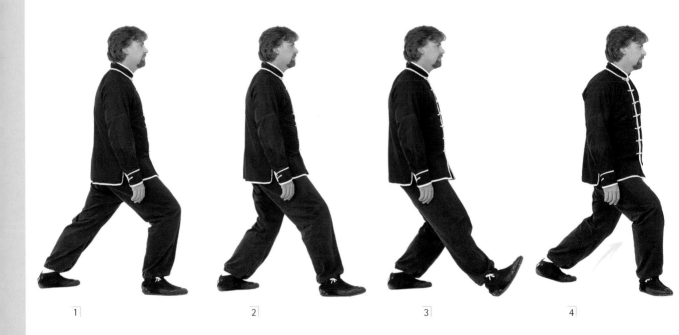

1   2   3   4

Repeat the exercise, beginning with the left foot forward and ending with a right forward stance.

The length of the forward stride is dictated by the amount of bend in the knee of the supporting leg. The less the bend, the shorter the stride. As your legs strengthen and you are able to bend your knees more, your stride will lengthen.

The head should not bob up and down as you move from stance to stance. It is important to look forwards and to maintain the same head height throughout the stepping process, keeping the head up in a natural position.

When you are familiar with the entire movement, add abdominal breathing. From the forward stance, breathe in when you lift your leg and through swivelling the foot, then breathe out for the rest of the movement.

Practise basic stepping as often as possible. Try not to move on to the next exercise until you are totally familiar with the stepping routine.

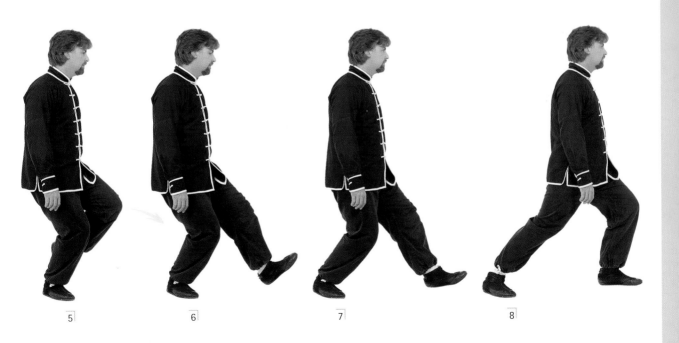

5   6   7   8

STEPPING - FORWARDS

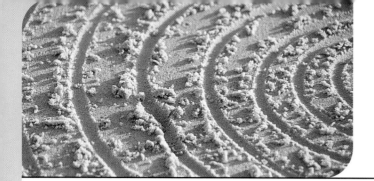

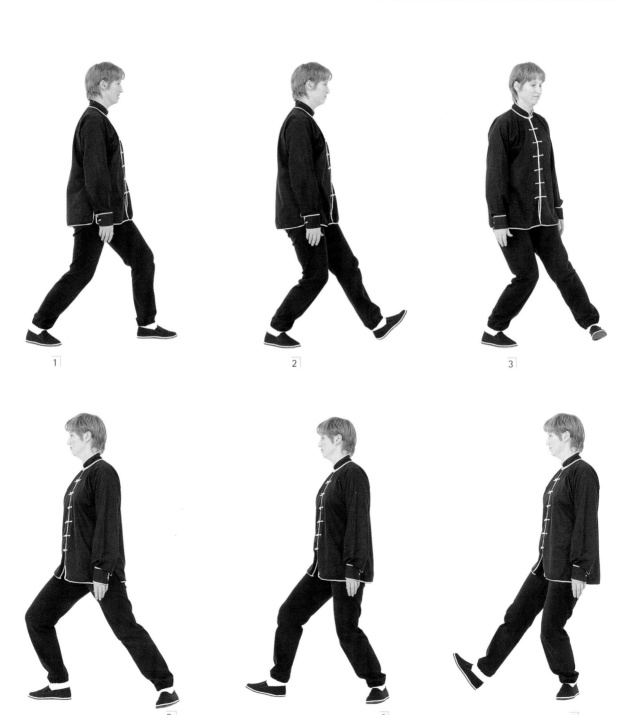

1

2

3

9

8

7

TURN
THROUGH 180 DEGREES

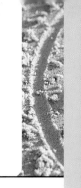

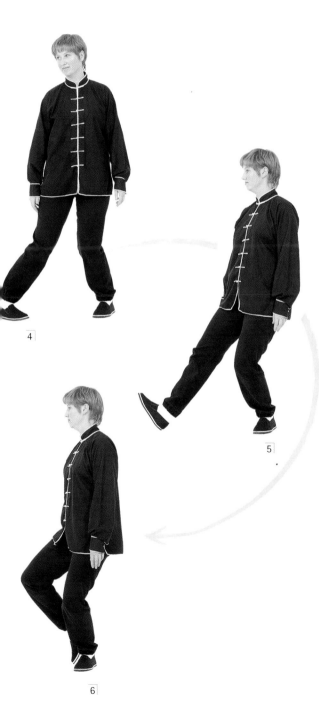

THIS *exercise adds the quality of turning while stepping, so the stepping routine can become an uninterrupted procedure.*

From a left forward stance (1), transfer the weight back (2), as if to take another step forwards but instead of swivelling the left foot outwards, swivel it inwards to 45 degrees (3). Place the left foot on the floor and transfer the weight onto it to bring you around 90 degrees to the right, with both feet pointed inward, flat on the floor (4). Continue transferring the weight to the left leg as you swivel the right foot on the heel, and end facing in the opposite direction (5).

Instead of transferring the weight forward, bring the right foot in and place it, toes pointing downward, next to the left ankle, making sure the knee is pointing straight forwards (6). The tips of the toes should touch the floor and the foot must be vertical. (This ensures that the next step won't be too narrow. If you turn and simply transfer the weight forwards into a right forward stance, and then bring the right foot back in a straight line, your right foot will touch the left, meaning that your stance is too narrow. You have to create the gap after the turn.)

From that position, extend the right leg forwards (7) and place the heel on the floor, marginally to the right. Remember that the heels must not be in a direct line with one another. Once the heel is correctly placed, transfer the weight to the right leg (8) and assume a right forward stance (9). Step into a left forward stance, then into another right forward stance. Repeat the exercise to the left.

Breathe out on the forward stance. Breathe in through the rock back and first part of the turn, then out through the rest of the turn, in as you bring the foot to the ankle, and out as you transfer the weight into the forward stance.

STEPPING - FORWARDS

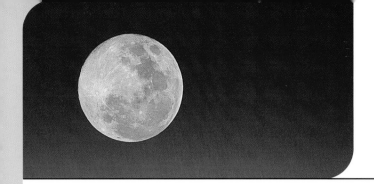

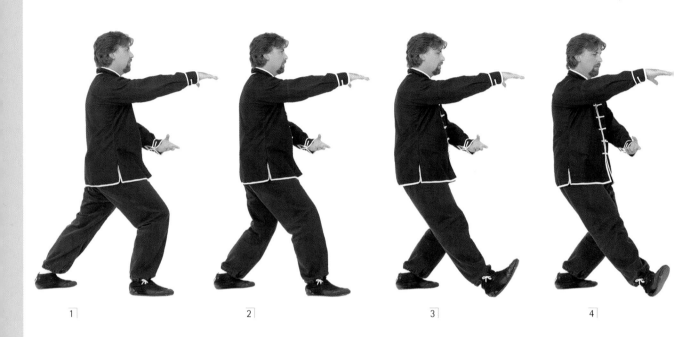

1

2

3

4

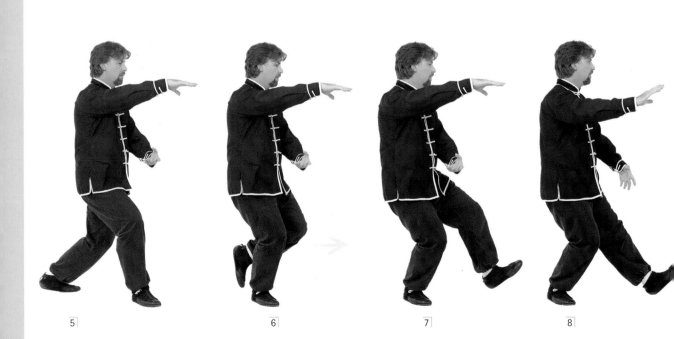

5

6

7

8

TAI CHI BALL

THIS *exercise is an introduction to learning to coordinate and move the entire body in a fluid relaxed manner, by adding the quality of arms to the basic stepping movement.*

Assume a right forward stance, and form the Tai Chi ball with right hand upper (1). Rock back, turn the right foot out, bring the left foot forwards and place the heel on the floor (2–8). The ball doesn't move while doing this. Transfer the weight into a left forward stance, while changing the ball to the left hand upper (9–11).

The ball only moves on the transfer of weight to the front foot. Ensure that you start the ball rolling when the weight begins to transfer, and finish exactly as you settle into the stance. Do not allow the hands to finish either before or after assuming the final stance; everything must stop at once. Repeat the process on the other side.

You can also add the ball to the turn and step *(see pages 58–59)*. Hold the ball on the rock back, through the turn, and on the withdrawal of the foot to next to the ankle. Place the foot out onto the heel and change as you shift forward into the forward stance. Simple and straightforward.

The breathing will not change from that suggested for the basic stepping procedure. The added arm movements should have no effect on the breathing at all.

Play with this exercise and be comfortable with it before moving onto the next stage, as it is important to develop coordination in the whole body.

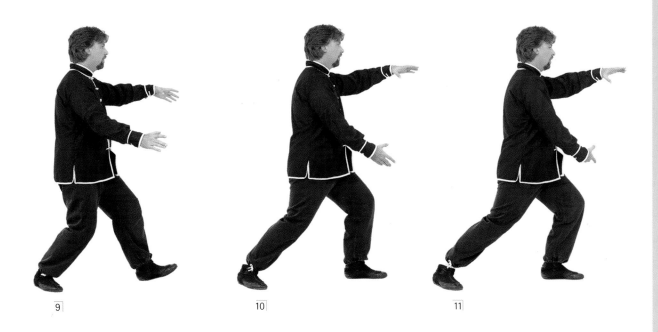

9 10 11

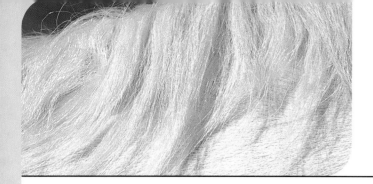

STEPPING - FORWARDS

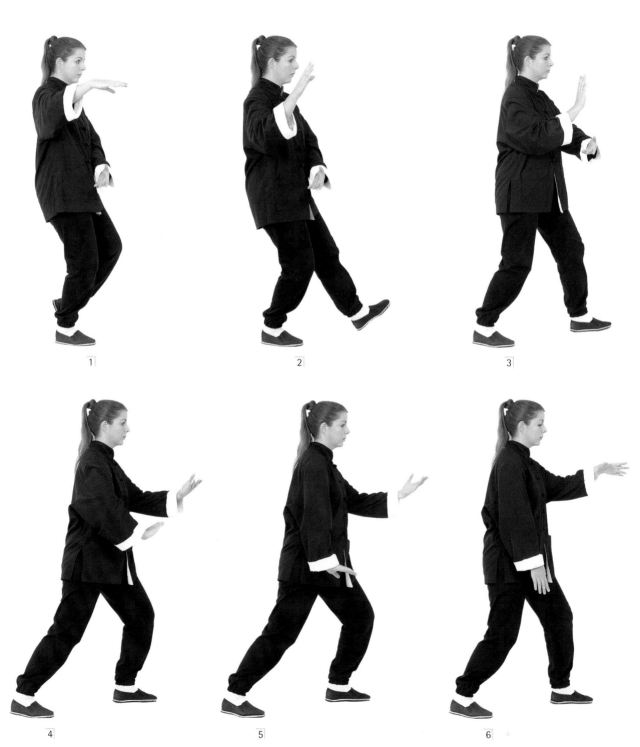

1

2

3

4

5

6

PARTING
WILD HORSE'S MANE

THIS *exercise continues working the entire body as one, except that we now add the quality of extension to the arms.*

Begin from an upright stance, weight on right leg and toes of left foot next to right ankle. Form the Tai Chi ball with the right hand uppermost (1). Step forward with left foot, heel first. As the weight transfers forward, instead of changing the Tai Chi ball, move the hands out into Parting Wild Horse's Mane (2–5). Hold this pose and ensure that the body is upright, as there is a tendency to lean forward slightly.

From Parting Wild Horse's Mane, form the hands back into the Tai Chi ball, this time with the left hand uppermost (6), as you rock back (7) and step (8–9) to repeat the exercise on the other side. Once again, ensure that all movement occurs on the transfer of weight forwards, and stops as the body settles into the forward stance.

The breathing sequence is the same as for basic stepping *(see page 57)*.

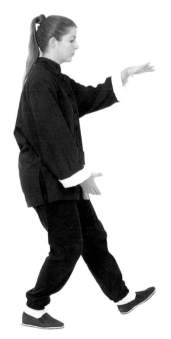

7

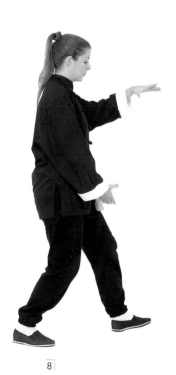

8

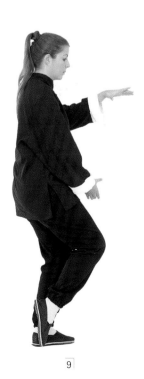

9

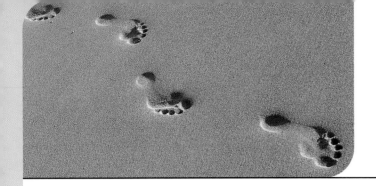

STEPPING - BACKWARDS

THIS *exercise introduces the element of stepping backwards in a straight line, and the correct transference of weight in a backward direction.*

Stand with the feet roughly 7cm (3in) apart, turn the left foot out to 45 degrees and bend the legs. Take the body weight on the left leg and slide the right foot forward until the leg is fully extended (1). Keep the foot flat on the floor, with all the weight on the left leg. Do not lean backwards, but maintain an erect posture. This is our starting point, also referred to as a back stance.

Keeping the weight on the left leg, gently swing the right leg round and backwards in a relaxed circular manner (2).

Place first the toes on the floor (3), then the ball of the foot (4), and lastly the heel, as you gently transfer the weight backwards onto the right foot (5), which should point outward at a 45-degree angle. Ensure the feet are not directly in line with each other, only the backs of the heels should line up. The left foot faces forward, still turned outward (6).

Once the weight is comfortably transferred to the right leg, turn the left foot to point straight forward by swivelling on the ball of the foot. This ensures that the feet are in a balanced position. If you swivel the foot straight from the heel, the feet will be lined up too directly, and your stance will be too narrow. Check the stance by bringing the left foot

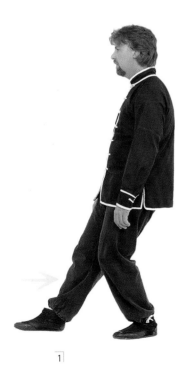

1

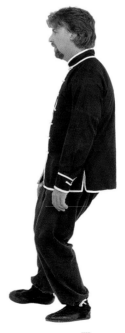

2

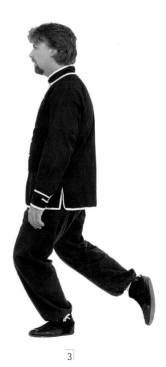

3

straight backwards. If the heels touch, then the stance is too narrow; if there is a gap of 5–7cm (2–3in) between the heels, the stance will be right.

Transfer your weight straight backwards by shifting from the hips (ensure that you do not lean while transferring). There should be no weight on the forward leg after the transfer, although there is an illusion of weight, as the foot is flat on the floor. Hips to shoulders should face forwards throughout the transfer of weight.

If one has been stepping forward, changing to a back stance is a simple transfer of weight backwards onto the back leg. However, to move from stepping backwards to stepping forwards again, one must bring the front foot back to the heel of the rear foot and then step forwards onto the heel. This is the same procedure as for turning through 180 degrees.

To step backwards with the Tai Chi ball, assume a back stance with left foot forward, form the ball with left hand uppermost. Hold the ball throughout the first step and swing, then change the ball when you transfer the weight and adjust the front foot.

Finally, breathe in on the first swing and step, and breathe out on the transfer and adjustment.

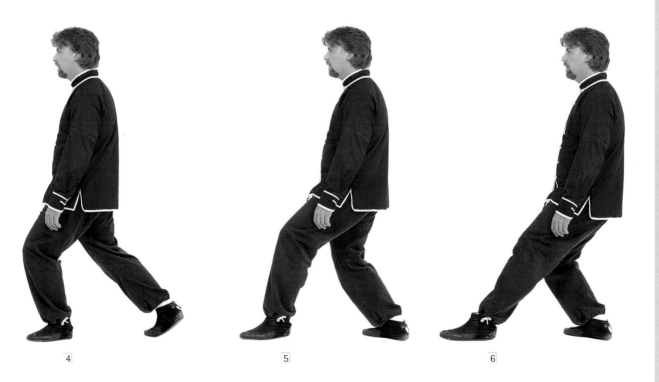

4   5   6

STEPPING - BACKWARDS

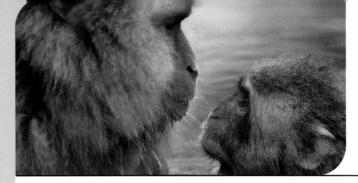

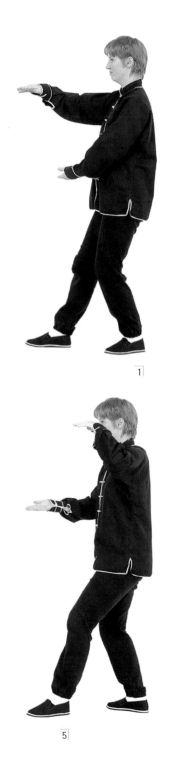

1

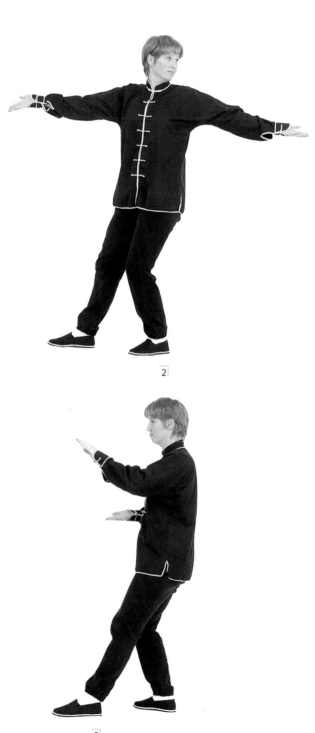

2

5

6

REPULSE MONKEY

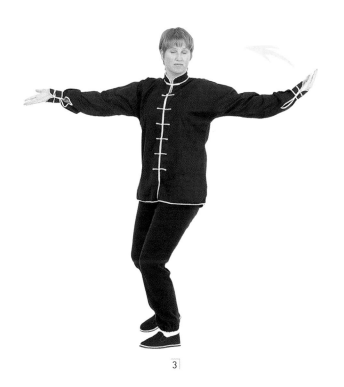

3

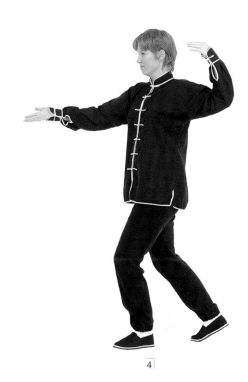

4

THIS *exercise adds the elements of arm movements and extension to backward stepping, and further helps to develop total body coordination.*

Assume a back stance, right foot forward, and form the Tai Chi ball with right hand uppermost (1). The first half of Repulse Monkey is done from the back stance. Turn the upper torso through 90 degrees to face left, while extending the arms to the back and front and glancing back at the left hand (2). Bend the left wrist and look forward (3), completing the Repulse Monkey movement throughout the sequence of stepping backwards (4), at the same time transferring the

weight and adjusting the front foot (5–6). This movement is slightly different from others, in that the arms move first, yet at the end everything must finish as one.

After you have completed the first Repulse Monkey with the backward step, you do not have to re-form the Tai Chi ball; you can flow into the next Repulse Monkey from where the hands stop.

The breathing changes somewhat with this exercise. The in-breath is done while the arms move through to the extension, and the out-breath is done through the step backwards, weight transfer and foot adjustment.

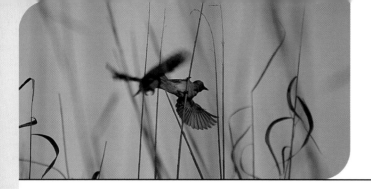

MOVEMENT ROUTINE

THIS short routine *(pages 68–73)*, is termed a run, or a short set, of movements. A run is usually practised in a continuous sequence, alternating left and right. A run may be static, in that it is done on one spot with very little foot movement, or it may involve taking a few steps in one direction that are then repeated in the opposite direction. Grasp Bird's Tail is a static run, alternating left and right, and gives us a sense of continuous unbroken movement and breathing.

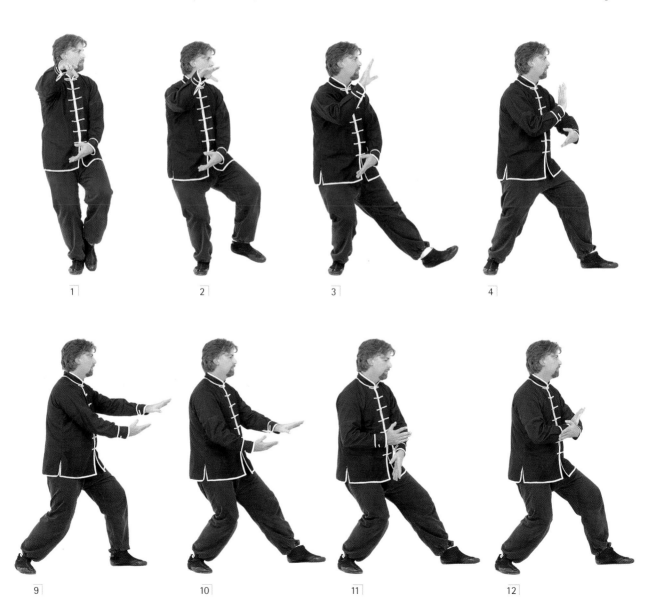

1   2   3   4

9   10   11   12

GRASP BIRD'S TAIL

Stand with the weight on the right leg, forming the Tai Chi ball, right hand upper (1). Step into a left forward stance, while raising the left forearm, wrist leading slightly, palm facing inward (2–4). Simultaneously drop the right hand and let it stop just below the left wrist, with the fingers upright, the palm facing forward and the fingertips about 5cm (2in) below the left wrist (5–6). Reach forward with the hands, but do not lean forward (7–8).

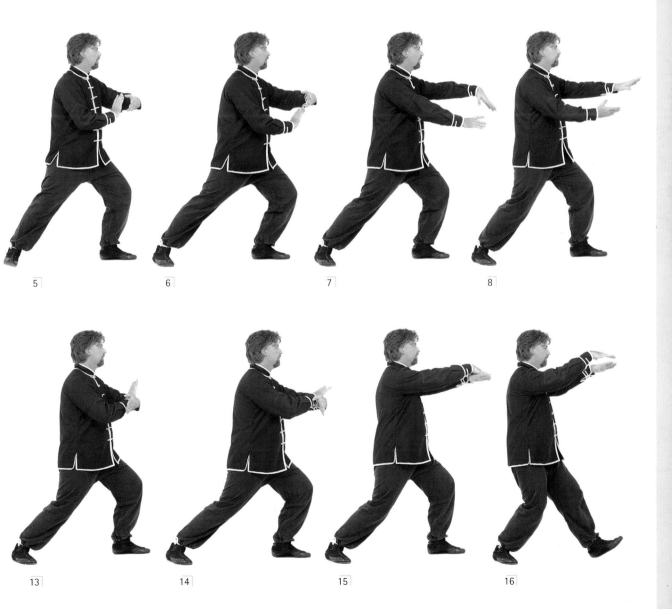

5

6

7

8

13

14

15

16

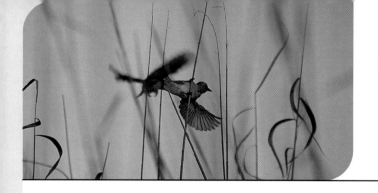

MOVEMENT ROUTINE
CONTINUED

Pull the hands backwards and downwards in a sinking motion, while transferring your weight backwards (9–10). Do not lean backward. Turn the left hand palm inward and place the palm of the right hand inside the left wrist, shifting the weight into a left forward stance (11–13). Turn the left palm to face down, while sliding the right palm over the back of the left wrist (14). Slowly extend the arms forwards while separating the hands and begin to rock backwards.

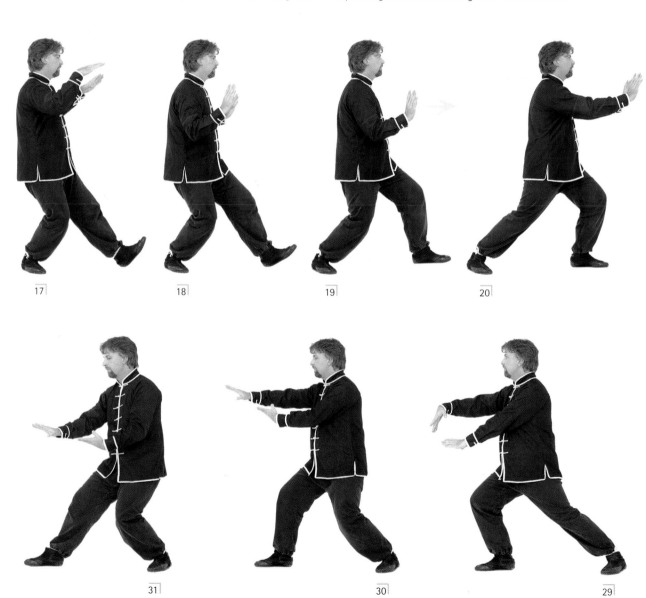

17　　18　　19　　20

31　　30　　29

GRASP BIRD'S TAIL

The hands separate and drift backwards towards the body as if they are sliding over the surface of a large ball (15–17). As the hands near the body, turn them as if you are about to push the ball forwards (18).

Push the ball forwards into a left forward stance, but do not lean forward (the weight shifts forwards from the hips [19–20], the torso does not lean forward). Leave the left hand where it is and circle the right hand upwards with the

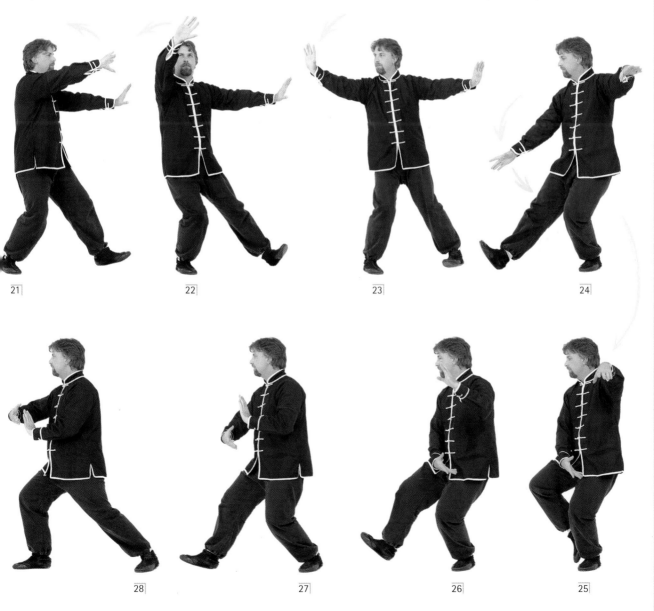

21

22

23

24

28

27

26

25

MOVEMENT ROUTINE
CONTINUED

palm facing out, while rocking back and turning the left foot inward through 180 degrees. The eyes should follow the hand, which should move in an arc without blocking your forward vision (21–23). Once the right hand drops below shoulder level, adjust the gaze forward again. All the weight should be on the left leg, with the right foot resting on the heel (24). Pull the right foot in as the right hand forms the bottom of the Tai Chi ball, with the left hand upper (25).

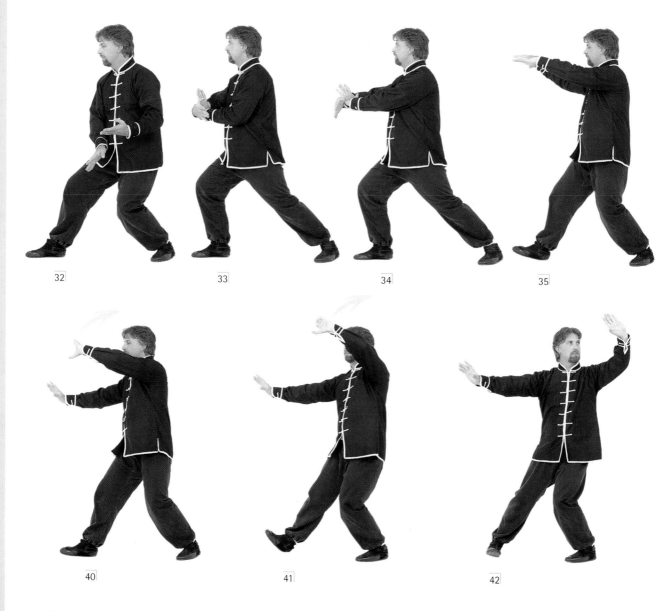

32

33

34

35

40

41

42

GRASP BIRD'S TAIL

Repeat the movement on the other side (26–45) until you return to the starting position (45 or 1).

When you are sure of the movements, include breathing. Breathe in on figure 1 and out through figures 2–6; in through 7–10, out through 11–13; breathe in through 14–17, out through 18–20; in through 21–25, out through 26–28; breathe in through 29–31, out through 32–33; in through 34–37, out through 38–39, and in through 40–45.

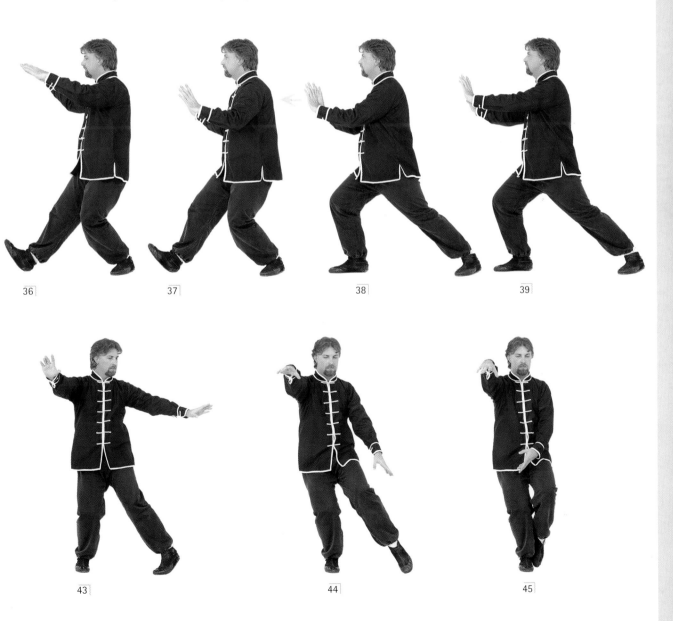

36

37

38

39

43

44

45

甜

The opponent doesn't know me:
I alone know him. To become a
peerless boxer results from this.
There are many boxing arts. Although
they use different forms, for the most
part, they don't go beyond the strong
oppressing the weak, and the slow
resigning to the swift.
The strong defeating the weak
and the slow hands ceding to swift
hands are all results of the physical
instinctive capacity and not of
well trained techniques.
From the sentence 'A force of four
ounces deflects a thousand pounds',
we know that the technique is not
accomplished with strength.
The spectacle of an old person
defeating a group of young people,
how can it be due to swiftness?
Wang Tsung-Yueh.

Tai Chi as a Martial Art

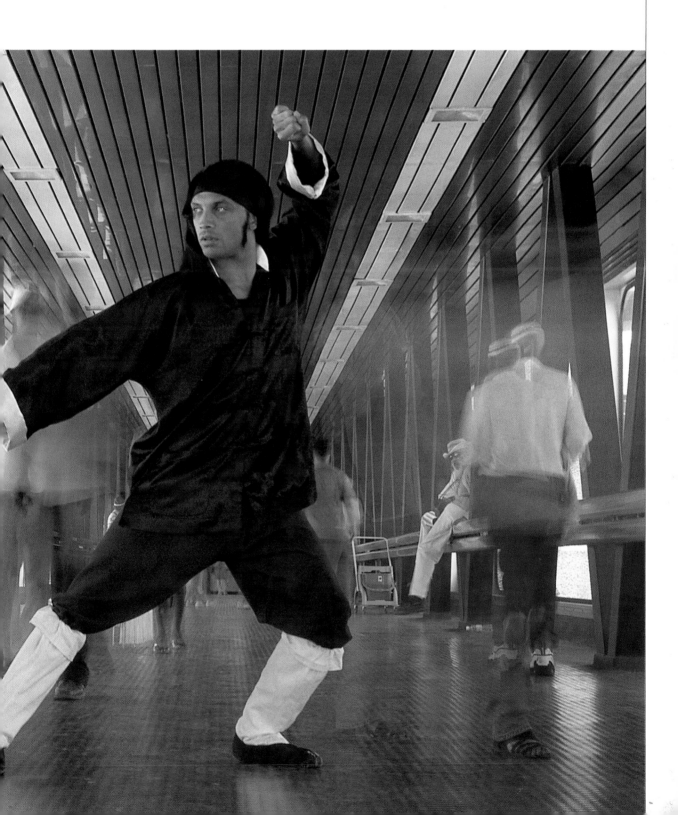

ACTING FROM INSTINCT

THE inevitable question, when one sees or hears about Tai Chi Chuan for the first time is: 'How can a discipline that is performed so slowly be used as a martial art?'

Tai Chi Chuan is performed slowly so that one can develop and perfect the techniques of movement. Through regular practice, we learn how the body flows from movement to movement, with only subtle changes of balance and control.

Balance and control give us a clearer understanding of the mechanics of our own body. Knowing this, we begin to understand the ways though which we can manoeuvre and disturb another person's body. This allows us to manipulate and control an opponent on a physical level.

Practising the forms in a relaxed manner teaches us how to relax. Physical relaxation leads to a calm state of mind, which allows the movements to sink into the subconscious.

Once something is subconscious it becomes instinctive. Instinctive actions are not guided by thought, therefore they are not vulnerable to emotions such as fear or uncertainty. Movement from instinct is controlled and fast.

There is no conscious thought being sent to the muscles prior to moving them, so the speed with which you react to a situation increases.

Through performing the movements of the Tai Chi forms, we gain a clearer understanding of our own body space

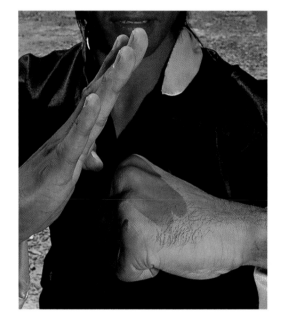

and the extension of our limbs, as well as of the space around us. This, in turn, enables us to have an increased sense of approaching danger (almost like an early warning system for the body). Heightened awareness reduces the shock value of a situation.

Shock has a powerful sedative effect on the mind. It disorientates us and freezes the conscious functions of the muscles. When this occurs,

instinct is the only thing that enables us to react. People react to emergency situations in relation to the degree of their knowledge of the circumstances. The greater the knowledge, the more effective the reaction. Tai Chi develops our understanding of our capabilities and, therefore, how we react.

To acquire the ability to act from instinct, and to gain the knowledge needed to practise Tai Chi Chuan as a martial art, requires discipline.

Practise every day if possible, twice a day if desired. During training, you need to concentrate on what you want to achieve and must not allow yourself to become distracted.

Tai Chi Chuan is neither a quick way to learn fighting skills, nor a short course in self defence. Rather, learning to use the martial arts aspects of Tai Chi is a lifelong commitment to something of immense value. Like all forms of martial arts, it takes many years of dedication and practice to become truly accomplished.

Above **Tai Chi's relaxed movements promote instinctive thought. In a crisis, if we do not think first, our reactions are faster and more effective.**

WORKING WITH A PARTNER

Most of our understanding of the martial arts aspects of Tai Chi Chuan comes from partner work. Working with a partner enables us to get the 'hands on' feel. It gets us over the fear of physical contact, allows us to develop a better sense of balance, and gives a clearer picture of what can happen if we are off centre.

Many people fear physical contact. They are uncertain and freeze up in a situation where contact is inevitable. If you want to be able to protect or defend yourself, it is important to reduce this fear. Partner work allows you to overcome this.

At advanced levels, free sparring is often a feature of training, allowing you to try out various techniques and movements. Sometimes punches or kicks make contact with the body. Getting used to the sensation of being hit is important, as it helps to reduce the shock of a genuine attack.

The majority of people are not exposed to violence in their daily lives. Feeling safe and secure creates a sense of complacency and comfort. But if something happens and we are suddenly confronted with a physically violent situation, we freeze. The mind refuses to accept what is happening and panic sets in. Training with a partner allows us to break this reaction.

Unlike some martial arts, which are predominantly linear, Tai Chi is based on circular movements and spirals. Therefore attacks are not met head on, and defence is not based solely on the athletic ability of the exponent.

Instead, defence is based on the relaxed nature of the individual. When we are relaxed, we can see situations with clarity. A relaxed calm mind is not clouded by negative emotions, so we think more clearly. When your body is relaxed, you can easily follow your opponent's moves, allowing you to counter them more easily.

When evaluating Tai Chi Chuan as a martial art, don't just look at the movements for their physical impact. You must also consider the underlying philosophy and values, as well as the principles that govern the movements and mechanics of the body.

Tai Chi Chuan as a martial art is not based on a single aspect – physical, mental or spiritual. It is only complete as a combination of them all.

Right **Young monks at the Shaolin Temple practise partner work. Getting used to being hit and to hitting back prepares one for conflict situations.**

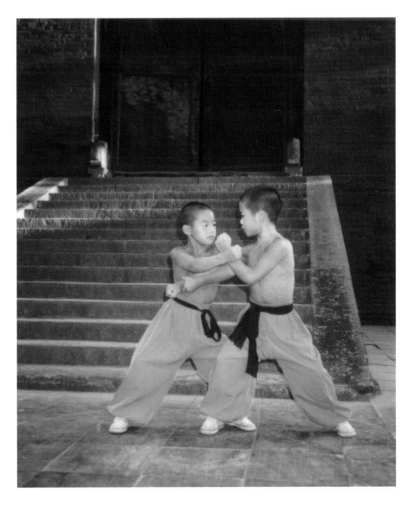

MECHANICS OF THE BODY

ALL MARTIAL arts are based on limited body movement. The intrinsic quality that defines martial arts in comparison with other sports is the optimum utilization of movement.

Body movement is not limitless, but is governed by the flexibility of each individual's muscles and joints. Most martial arts utilize one aspect more than others. Some disciplines use mainly the arms, while others rely more on leg techniques. However, all movement remains constrained by the limits imposed by the body.

As with the other martial arts, the movements and techniques used in Tai Chi Chuan are based on understanding the principles of the body's mechanics.

The legs are the body's 'long range' weapons. They are powerful and flexible with strong muscles and, if used correctly, can incapacitate or seriously injure an opponent. Lack of flexibility does not reduce their effectiveness, it only reduces their range of movement.

The legs' weakness is that they can generally only be used one at a time, and if trapped, open the groin area to attack. An injury to a leg affects the mobility of the individual.

The leg has two joints. The ankle is flexible, so it has a range of movement, but for a kick to be effective, the ankle is normally 'locked' into a particular position. The fragile ankle bone therefore becomes a target area.

The knee can only bend in one direction, so force exerted on the knee from the side or front will weaken it.

The muscles of the upper leg give lift and power. A muscle injury can reduce the range of movement and limit the leg's ability to support the body.

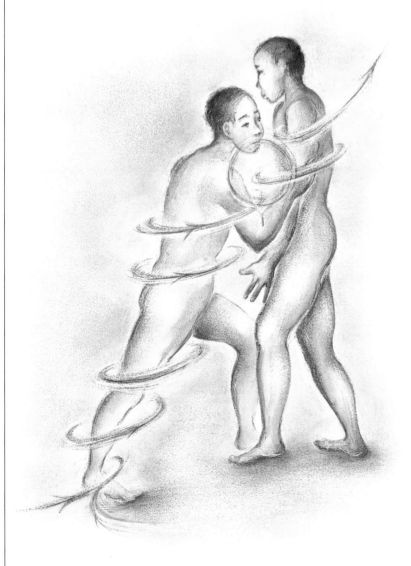

Left **The legs are the body's long range weapons; the arms are the medium range weapons; and the elbows and knees the short range weapons. By forcing your opponent to move in a circle, you deflect his attack.**

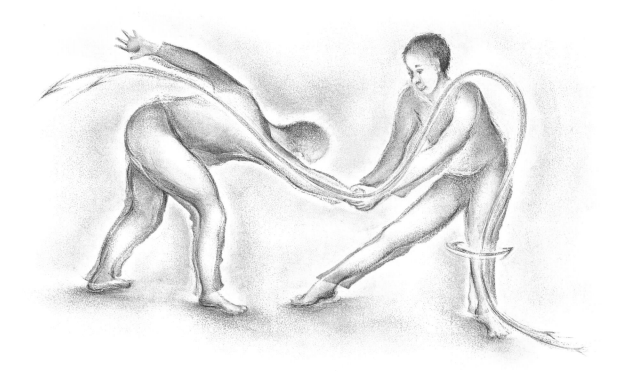

The arms are the 'medium range' weapons of the body. They are flexible, have a large range of movement, and can build up speed and power over a short distance. The arms can be used either singly or simultaneously. Their effectiveness lies in the alignment of the torso. If the torso is turned too far in any particular direction, the arms' effectiveness is largely reduced.

Although the wrist is flexible, it can be injured if it becomes trapped or if too much pressure is placed on it in a backward or a lateral direction. The elbow can only flex in one direction and pressure from the opposite direction can injure or break it.

The shoulder gives the arm freedom of movement, but becomes vulnerable if pressure is exerted from behind.

The 'short range' weapons are the elbows and knees, which consist largely of bone, with no protective muscle. They are capable of inflicting incapacitating damage, and are difficult to block or counter at close range.

Tai Chi Chuan employs the concept of a circle to establish a defence or attack. This means constantly moving around your opponent, while avoiding any attacks in a linear direction. By forcing your opponent to keep moving in a circle, you restrict his movements.

Attacks are deflected in a way that compels your opponent to turn even further, thereby exposing the side or back of his body.

Tai Chi Chuan is seldom competitive, so there are few rules to limit technique or govern strikes. Partner work in class allows one to experiment with the various techniques in a safe, controlled manner. Regular practice gives us a better understanding of the mechanics of our own body, while partner work helps us to understand the manipulation of those mechanics in an attack or defence situation.

Above When the opponent is hard, I am soft – this is called *tsou,* or yielding. When I follow the opponent and he becomes backed up, it is called *mien,* or adherence. If the opponent's movement is quick, then quickly respond; if his movement is slow, then follow slowly. Although the changes are numerous, the principle that pervades them is only one.

Wang Tsung-Yueh

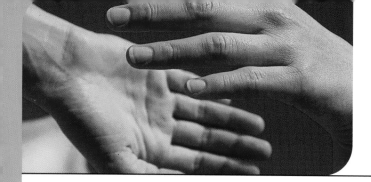

PARTNER WORK

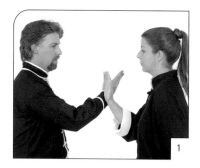

1

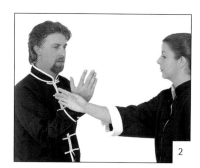

2

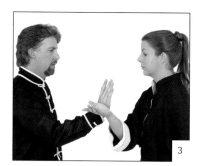

3

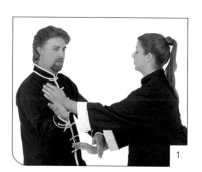

1

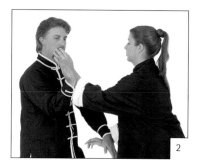

2

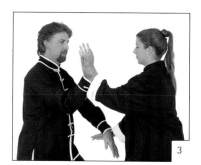

3

PUSHING HANDS is a movement routine for two people. It introduces the practice of remaining in contact with an opponent, promotes interaction, develops a sense of balance, and teaches us to manipulate an opponent's energy. At advanced levels it develops the principle of manipulating your opponent's energy for the purpose of defence.

The initial exercises for Pushing Hands are single arm movements (1-4 top), which progress into movements using both arms (1-6 bottom). These are then added to stepping routines and, once they are mastered, free movement is introduced.

In the early stages, the pace is steady and rhythmic. Once you are familiar with the double arm and step routines you learn to speed them up. When free movement is introduced, the idea is to increase the pace to the point of simulating actual combat speed, while remaining in contact with your opponent as much as possible.

This concept of remaining in contact with an opponent is known as *Chi Sao,* or sticking hands. *Chi Sao* techniques are incorporated into many other styles of Chinese martial arts, the best-known being *Wing Chun.*

PUSHING HANDS

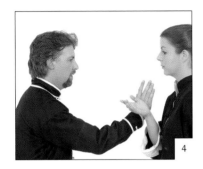

4

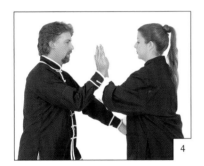

4

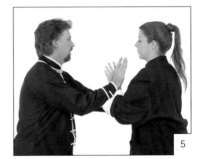

5

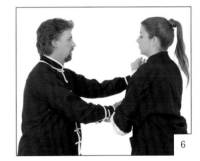

6

Pushing Hands is a variation on the concept of *Chi Sao*. The basic intention of *Chi Sao* is to develop sensitivity in the arms through constant contact and movement with an opponent, which allows us to become sensitive to another person's movements.

By 'feeling' an opponent's movements, we can learn to judge his intention and ascertain the direction that his next move will take. This enables us to counter with ease, and helps us to manipulate our opponent into a position of weakness and vulnerability.

It is not unheard of for very advanced practitioners of Tai Chi Chuan to be able to judge an opponent's intention from the lightest of hand contact.

There is a legend of two masters who challenged each other to a match. They took up their fighting postures and their forward hands touched. There they stood, completely still with only the slightest contact between their hands. Time passed and eventually they broke apart and shook hands. When asked why they did not actually move or fight, the reply was: 'Neither of us could find an opening'.

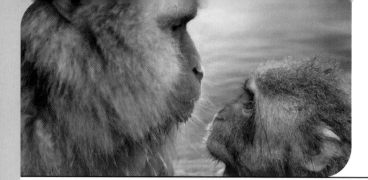

SELF-DEFENCE

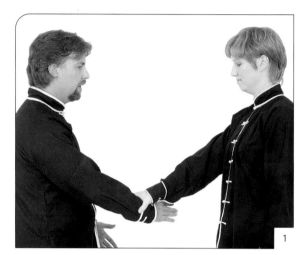

Defender   Attacker

WORKING with a partner means taking movements you have already learned and applying them in a specific manner. These pages show two very simple movements which involve the application of Repulse Monkey *(see pages 50–51)*. They both involve the hand being grabbed by an opponent (1).

Although Repulse Monkey is normally used in conjunction with a backward stepping motion, it is important to realize the possibilities available for self-defence if one is grabbed or pulled by the wrist.

The first movement (shown on this page) demonstrates the defender's forward hand being grabbed. He then withdraws

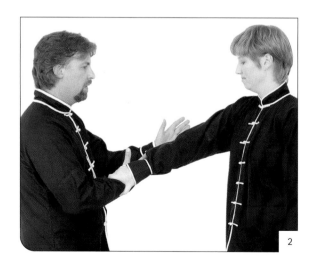

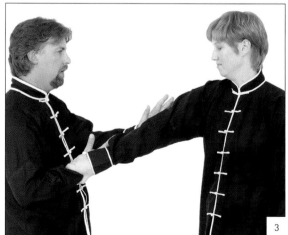

REPULSE MONKEY

it, turning the palm upwards (2). This twists the opponent's arm and allows the defender to strike towards the elbow of the opponent's arm (3).

The second self defence movement based on Repulse Monkey (shown below) also works off the hand being grabbed (1). This time, however, instead of striking towards the attacker's elbow, the defender thrusts his flat hand straight forward into his opponent's face (2).

This movement works with even more effect if, after your opponent grabs your hand, he or she is then foolish enough to pull you forward towards him- or herself.

When working in a Tai Chi class situation, the object of the exercise is to familiarize oneself with the sensation of being grabbed, so that the response to an attack on the respective target areas can become a natural action. Often students will rotate with one another to experience working with opponents of different strengths and heights.

As defensive techniques, the first exercise can seriously damage the elbow region, while the second could result in a broken nose, with the addition of whiplash to the neck area. When you work with a partner in training, take the greatest care to prevent any injury to yourself or your partner.

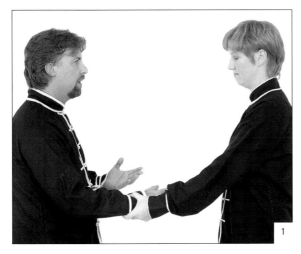

Defender   Attacker

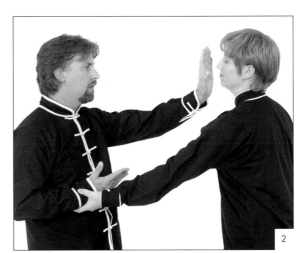

ATTACK

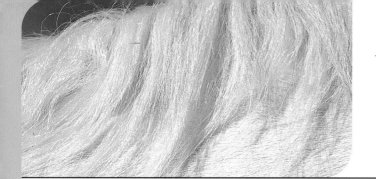

THESE *illustrations depict two variations to an application for Parting Wild Horse's Mane (pages 46-47). They are taken from the starting position of a pre-fight posture, which is almost identical to a back stance.*

The first variation (1–3 top) shows what takes place when an opponent throws a punch at you. The back of one hand and arm block the move, while the other hand sweeps upward and makes contact with the attacker's face, either on the cheekbone, under the eye or against the temple. As this is done, the defender's stance changes from a back stance to a forward stance, adding momentum to the application.

In the second variation (1–3 bottom); instead of blocking as the attacker punches, the defender lifts her arms to make contact with her opponent's arm from underneath. A small step to the side moves the defender to the attacker's side and, with the forward arm extended up and out, the elbow can make close contact with the opponent's armpit. The defender's arm is extended while assuming a forward stance, and if a slight twist is added to the torso, her opponent will be lifted slightly off balance.

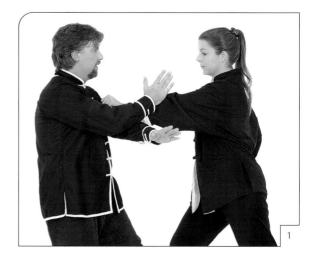

Defender   Attacker

CAUTIONARY

Both applications depicted can cause injury to the head or spine. They are shown simply as examples of the many possibilities available for attack, but readers are cautioned not to attempt them without proper instruction and training beforehand.

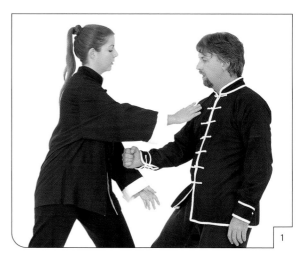

Defender   Attacker

PARTING
WILD HORSE'S MANE

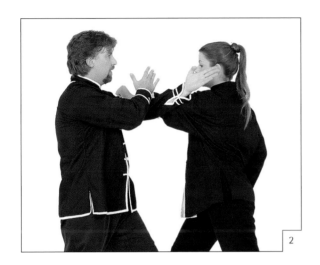

2

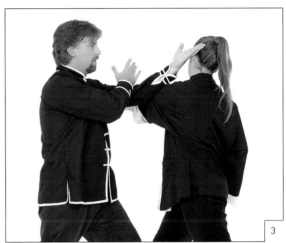

3

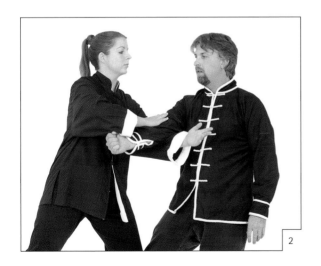

2

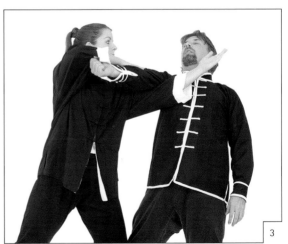

3

TAI CHI CHUAN *is not only a series of exercise routines, nor is it only a martial art. It is a combination of both which amalgamates into a process by which you can live life to the full, a process that will allow you to maintain an above-average level of health and vitality well into old age.*

Whenever we start any new form of exercise or sport, it is important to determine its worth to ourselves. Some of the questions one tends to ask include 'what can it offer me, what are the pros and cons of participation, what are the long-term results, and what are the advantages?' The following section attempts to answer some of them with regard to Tai Chi Chuan.

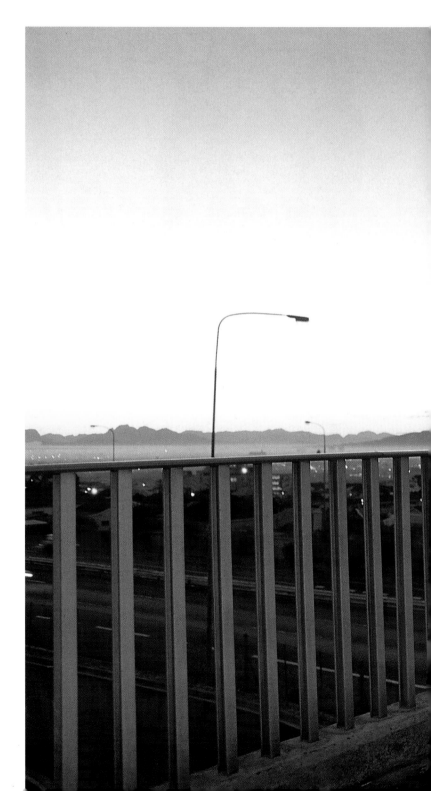

BENEFITS OF TAI CHI

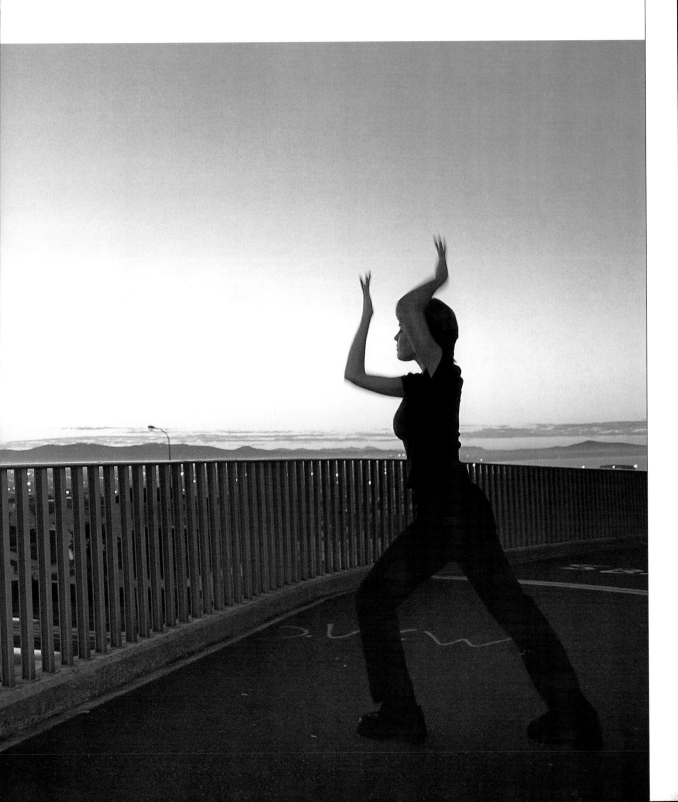

POSTURE, JOINTS AND MUSCLES

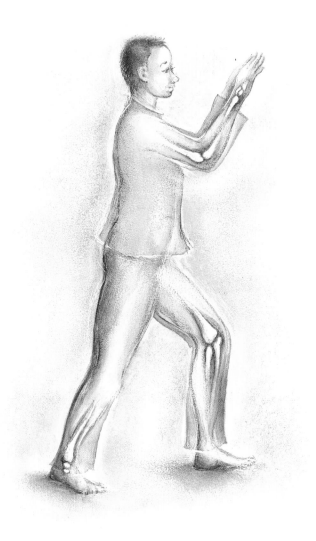

regular practice, maintaining the correct posture ceases to be a conscious thought, and we begin to adjust our posture to that which has become familiar and comfortable.

When we improve our posture, we reduce the chance of developing back problems and alleviate the discomfort of existing problems.

Regular Tai Chi practice trains us to improve and maintain our posture while enhancing the body's freedom of movement.

JOINTS

One of the first conditions to afflict the body as it ages is a stiffening of the joints, which gradually lose their range of movement, making it harder to move comfortably.

In Tai Chi Chuan, all the major joints are utilized in a gentle manner. The ankle, knee and hip are used to move the legs. The torso moves in a circular manner that allows the spinal column to have a certain amount of torque, or rotation. The entire arm is used, from the shoulder through the elbow and into the wrists.

Above **As you progress, your joints and muscles will become toned, flexible and stronger.**

POSTURE

Many people suffer posture-related problems that are caused by sitting at a desk for too long or from moving incorrectly in physically oriented jobs.

One of the first things learned in Tai Chi Chuan is how to stand correctly. Having the correct stance ensures that body weight is distributed evenly on both legs. Once we can comfortably assume the correct stance, we can concentrate on holding our bodies in an erect manner, while ensuring that our stance is relaxed. Next we learn to maintain this posture while stepping forwards or backwards.

Arm movements are introduced and slowly we acclimatize the body and mind to maintaining an erect posture in both stillness and movement. With

In many contact sports, such as rugby and American football, joint-related injuries can prevent sportsmen from participating in their chosen sport, and limit participation in other sports. However, while injuries or physical disabilities may preclude people from participating in many sports, they do not prevent the practice of Tai Chi.

With a little effort, one can learn to utilize to the full whatever movement is available, strengthening joints over time and leading to the possibility of further movement.

Lack of knowledge of alternatives often prevents people from maintaining their health after sustaining an injury. Tai Chi's low impact movements limit the potential for injury and help to strengthen, rather than weaken, joints. The chance of developing joint-related conditions such as arthritis or rheumatism is reduced, and sufferers often find the associated discomfort is alleviated through Tai Chi.

Muscles

The joints allow the limbs to move, but it is the muscles that give control, strength and power to movement.

Sporting activity is governed by the way in which we condition (train) our muscles. This can take various forms, including training with weights. Poor conditioning can lead to muscle tissue being damaged. If too much damage is done, an injury could become a permanent hindrance to correctly performing that particular activity.

Muscle-related injuries are often the result of incorrect posture in an activity, over-extension of a muscle, or exerting pressure on a muscle before it is warmed up sufficiently. Tai Chi Chuan helps prevent injury to muscles caused by these conditions.

Posture-related muscle injuries are eliminated as a result of adhering to the correct posture at all times. Over-extension leads to imbalanced posture and a weakness of stance, so there is

no risk of over-extending the muscles if one maintains the correct posture.

The slow, rhythmic nature of the movements allows muscles to warm up comfortably and safely. Even if one neglects the warm-up exercises, the chance of injuring muscles is reduced. (Remember that it is only reduced, not prevented altogether. No matter how light the exercise, one should always warm up properly beforehand.)

As one grows older, the risk of injury to muscles increases in proportion to the vigorous nature of the activity. However with regular practice, muscles are strengthened and toned. The open, sometimes low, movements of Tai Chi allow muscles to stretch and maintain flexibility, while the steady relaxed pace reduces the risk of injury. This allows one to practise well into old age, with little risk of injury.

Tai Chi Chuan does not focus on one group of muscles more than others. Yes, the legs do more work than the upper body, but they have to support the body's weight comfortably.

Regular martial arts practice builds the body naturally. If you are carrying excess weight, you will tone down, and if you are young and still developing, you will build your body up to what it should be.

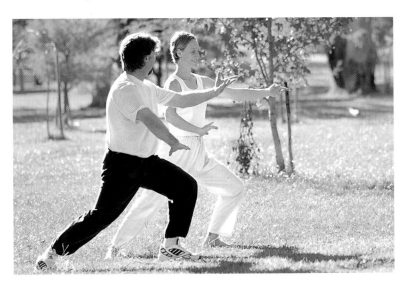

Left **Athletes recovering from muscle-related injuries can get back into condition by using Tai Chi exercises.**

CARDIOVASCULAR SYSTEM

HOUSED within our bodies lies an extensive system of veins, arteries and capillaries. This entire system is connected to one fairly small muscle, the heart. Roughly the size of a man's clenched fist, the heart performs an incredible job of pumping blood through the body. Yet, as with any item of equipment that functions nonstop hour after hour, day after day, the heart is vulnerable to failure. Among the most common causes of cardiovascular disease are high blood pressure, high cholesterol levels, stress, smoking and circulatory malfunction.

Blood pressure is the force that blood exerts on the inside walls of the blood vessels. It is measured in the same manner as atmospheric pressure (that is the height to which a column of mercury in a measuring tube will rise). Our blood pressure rises and falls with each heartbeat. It is highest as the heart contracts (about 120mm of mercury) and lowest as the heart relaxes (about 80mm of mercury). This is expressed medically as 120 over 80, or 120/80.

Normal blood pressure fluctuates throughout the day, dropping while we are sleeping or resting, and rising during periods of activity or stress (sometimes to dangerous levels, depending on the circumstances). Low blood pressure causes few problems, unless one is driving a car or operating heavy machinery, as it can lead to episodes of dizziness or faintness.

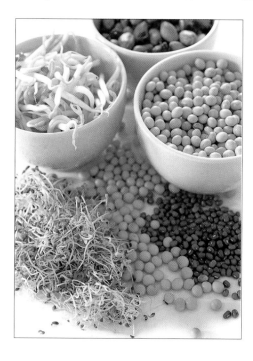

Smoking promotes a disorder known as atherosclerosis, which falls into a category known as arteriosclerosis, or hardening of the arteries. This happens naturally with the ageing process, but smoking speeds it up to dangerous levels. Hardening makes the arteries brittle, and any undue pressure on the inside can cause a rupture in the artery (somewhat like a garden hose left out in the sun, that becomes brittle and starts to leak when the tap is turned on).

High cholesterol, which also falls into the category of arteriosclerosis, is enhanced by the consumption of foods with a higher than average fat content. Cholesterol is produced naturally by the liver and flows through the bloodstream. Because it already exists in the body, excessive amounts of fatty foods overload the system. The added cholesterol floods the bloodstream and the excess becomes deposited on artery walls, including those in the heart and brain. These deposits narrow the diameter of the arteries, preventing the free flow of blood and increasing blood pressure. If this narrowing becomes a total blockage, it can cause a heart attack or stroke.

Stress, which causes blood pressure to rise dangerously, is an indirect cause of cardiovascular disease. The origins of stress can be physical, through reduced movement or a lack of exercise; or mental, such as loss, bereavement, retrenchment or anger. However, most stress-related disease results from years of accumulated problems and worries all manifesting at once. This makes the diagnosis very hard from a medical viewpoint. Daily lifestyle has a lot to do with stress. Long working hours, irregular sleeping patterns, lack of regular exercise, overindulgence in alcohol or drugs, and many other factors add up over the years and take their toll.

Circulatory malfunction is usually caused by a blockage in a vein or artery. The blockage is normally due to fatty deposits that break away from the walls of the veins or arteries and become lodged in a narrow section, or an intersection of two smaller veins. Veins have one-way valves which only allow blood to flow in one direction. If a vein is blocked by a foreign object, it upsets the flow and the pressure behind the blockage increases.

The nature of the steady rhythmic movements of Tai Chi Chuan will not shock the cardiovascular system. The increased body movements are done at a pace that the cardiovascular system can adjust to safely. The gentle increase ensures that the optimum amount of blood flows to the muscles,

Left Pulses, sprouts and grains are low in saturated fats and can therefore, as part of a natural healthy diet, help to prevent cardiovascular disease.

Right There are no age barriers in Tai Chi, and performing the exercises on a regular basis benefits the elderly by keeping them mobile and supple.

providing them with the right amount of oxygen, proteins, carbohydrates and fats. Muscle fatigue during exercise is a sign that the muscles are not being provided with the correct quantities of nutrients and the blood is flowing through them so quickly that they are unable to extract what is needed.

As the pace of exercise increases, the heart rate increases, triggering warning signals if there is the risk of over-exertion. Tai Chi allows the heart to adjust comfortably; being a muscle, this gentle adjustment on a regular basis has a strengthening affect.

As body movement increases, the muscles require more energy. This comes from using excess stored fats, thereby lowering the levels in the body. This in turn slows the build-up of deposits in the arteries. With the

blood flowing more quickly, the veins and arteries start to regain their former elasticity, reducing hardening. As pressure on the inner walls is reduced, the blood pressure is lowered.

As the body relaxes, mental stresses also ease. To perform Tai Chi Chuan correctly takes concentration, and the break from focusing on our worries often affords us a clearer picture of the problem. When we come back to it, we may even find a solution.

When practised regularly, Tai Chi Chuan develops a strong cardiovascular system in young people, limiting the potential for problems later in life. In the middle to elderly age groups, the cardiovascular system is strengthened gradually, allowing the body to adjust and reducing the chance of problems occurring through over-exertion.

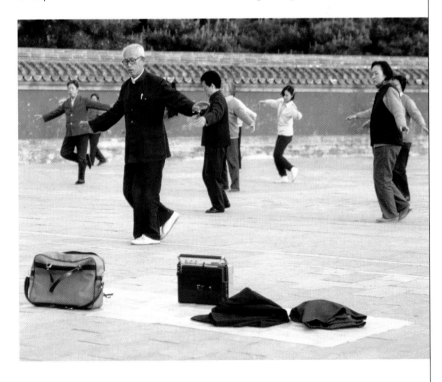

PROMOTING WELLBEING

THROUGH the practice of Tai Chi Chuan, we learn to develop and utilize the method of breathing known as abdominal breathing. This ensures that the lungs are being put to full use and that they can take in the maximum volume of air with each breath. This, in turn, translates into a greater supply of oxygen to the body.

The lungs contain millions of fine vessels called capillaries, through which the body's entire blood supply passes about once a minute. Correct breathing ensures that the body is supplied with sufficient oxygen.

The brain uses about 20 per cent of the oxygen we breathe and about 15 per cent of the body's blood supply. Blood passes through, and is filtered by, the kidneys approximately every four minutes. It is clear, therefore, that the internal organs of the body will benefit from any increase in oxygen.

Tai Chi Chuan is beneficial to the entire body – external and internal, as it promotes physical, emotional and mental wellbeing.

It tones, strengthens and increases muscle and joint flexibility and, as it is low impact in nature, there is no undue pressure placed on the joints. Tai Chi allows the cardiovascular system to safely build up in pace with little risk. It improves balance and coordination and participation is not limited by age or weight. The risk of injury is negligible, so it is safe to continue exercising while recovering from a physical injury. It can be followed comfortably throughout pregnancy, and women who practise Tai Chi at this time frequently report an absence of pre- and post-natal problems.

Tai Chi Chuan can be practised more than once a day with no risk of over-exertion, and requires only a small amount of space at first.

Formal classes are generally geared towards developing sufficient skill to enable you to practise independently as soon as possible. Later on, you can practise with a partner or in a group.

As our ability to perform Tai Chi Chuan improves and we become healthier, our posture is corrected and we begin to breathe more effectively. With this comes the sensation of feeling better about ourselves, which leads to an increase in confidence and vitality, and an improvement in our own lives, which begins to rub off on those around us, so that we improve the quality of their lives as well.

Right **Sound health and wellbeing are among the long-term benefits of Tai Chi Chuan, leading to greater personal growth and a positive outlook.**

Retaining Integrity

Whilst cultivating creativity,
also cultivate receptivity.
Retain the mind like that of a child,
which flows like running water.

When considering any thing,
do not lose its opposite.
When thinking of the infinite,
do not forget infinity.

Act with honour,
but retain humility.
By acting according to the way of
the Tao, set others an example.

By retaining the integrity of the
inner and external worlds,
true selfhood is maintained,
and the inner world made fertile.

Lao Tzu

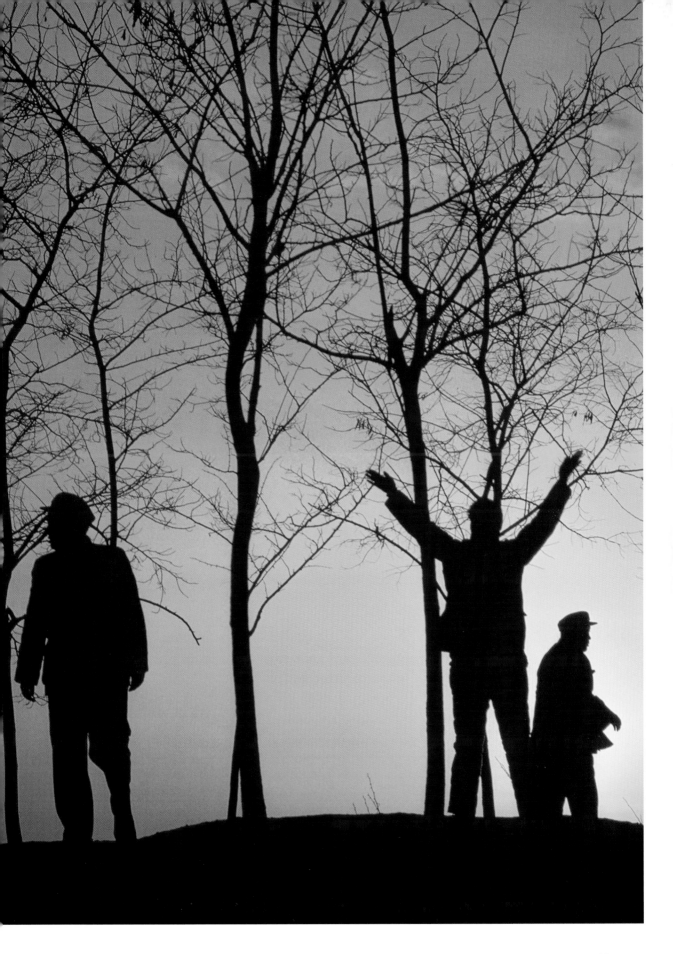

Contacts

As Tai Chi is not a competitive sport, there is no overall governing body. For information on Tai Chi classes in your area, try the Yellow Pages, your local sports council, or the societies and associations listed below.

INTERNATIONAL TAIJIQUAN & SHAOLIN WUSHU ASSOCIATION (ITSWA)
- Sifu Derek Frearson
- 28 Linden Farm Drive,
- Countesthorpe, Leicester LE8 5SX
- Tel/fax: (116) 277-4260
- email: Sifu@itswahq.freeserve.co.uk
- www.itswa.freeserve.co.uk

INTERNATIONAL TAOIST TAI CHI SOCIETY
Europe:
- Bounstead Road, Blackheath,
- Colchester, Essex CO2 0DE UK
- Tel: (1206) 576167
- Fax: (1206) 572269
- email: europe@ttcs.org
USA:
- 1310 North Monroe Street,
- Tallahassee, Florida 32303
- Tel: (850) 224-5438
- email: usa@ttcs.org
Australia:
- 75 Riverside Road,
- East Fremantle, WA 6158
- PO Box 23 Palmyra WA 6157
- Tel/fax: (8) 9339-1331
- email: australia@ttcs.org

INTERNATIONAL YANG STYLE TAI CHI CHUAN ASSOCIATION
USA:
- 280 Newport Way, NW#B14,
- Issaquah, WA 98027
- Tel/fax: (425) 369-8841
Europe:
- Valhallavagen 58,
- 11427 Stockholm, Sweden
- Tel: (8) 201-800
- Fax: (8) 201-832
China:
- No.10 Wu Cheng West Street,
- Taiyuan, Shanxi, PRC 03006
- Tel: (351) 704-2713

UK AND IRELAND
BRITISH COUNCIL FOR THE CHINESE MARTIAL ARTS (BCCMA)
- c/o 110 Frensham Drive,
- Stockingford, Nuneaton,
- Warwickshire CV10 9QL
- Tel/fax: (906) 302-1036
- email: info@bccma.demon.uk
- www.bccma.org.uk

TAI CHI UNION FOR GREAT BRITAIN
- 1 Littlemill Drive, Balmoral Gardens,
- Crookston, Glasgow G53 7GE
- Tel: (141) 810-3482
- Fax: (141) 810-3741
- email: secretary@taichiunion.com

EUROPE
EUROPEAN WUSHU FEDERATION (EWF)
- 11 Lucas Close, Yatchley,
- Camberly GU17 7JO
- United Kingdom

CHINA
INTERNATIONAL WUSHU FEDERATION (IWUF)
- 3 Anding Road, Chaoyang District,
- Beijing 100101

USA
USA WUSHU KUNGFU FEDERATION (USAWKF)
- 6313 Harford Road,
- Baltimore, Maryland 21214
- Tel: (410) 444-6666
- Fax: (410) 426-5524

NEW ZEALAND
NEW ZEALAND WUSHU FEDERATION
- 74 May Road, Mt Roskill, Auckland
- Tel: (9) 309-2855
- Fax: (9) 309-6760

SOUTH AFRICA
CHINESE MARTIAL ARTS AND HEALTH CENTRE (CMAHC)
- 85 Station Rd, Observatory, Cape Town
- Tel: (21) 448-2594
- email: cmahc@mweb.co.za
- www.cmahc.co.za

INDEX

ACKNOWLEDGEMENTS

The author wishes to thank the following people whose assistance was instrumental in making this book happen: My teachers and students, who gave me the reason; Corinne, for the opportunity; Lauren and Lille, two talented students, for their patience during the photo shoots; Ryno, for his professionalism; my friends, Bille Lee, John, Cathy, Karl and Catherine for their support and encouragement; and Sheryl, Claire and Gill at New Holland for their help and suggestions.

The publishers would like to thank Nick Aldridge and Alzette Prins for their patience and unfailing enthusiasm; calligrapher Simon Spiller for adding a unique touch with his interpretive brushstrokes. Models Deirdre Rhodes, Annaline DeWit, Sifu Luke Skywalker and Philip Coetzee for their kind assistance with the photoshoot.

PHOTOGRAPHIC CREDITS

All photography by Ryno Reyneke, with the exception of those supplied by the following photographers and/or agencies (copyright rests with these individuals and/or their agencies): NHIL = New Holland Image Library

2-3	Nicholas Aldridge	15	Nicholas Aldridge	48 (top)	Gallo Images
4	Nicholas Aldridge	16	Corbis Images	54 (top)	Nicholas Aldridge
7a	Nicholas Aldridge	24	Colin Lewis	58 (top)	Nicholas Aldridge
7b	Nicholas Aldridge	25	Peter Baasch	68 (top)	Nicholas Aldridge
7c	Nicholas Aldridge	35	Nicholas Aldridge	75	Nicholas Aldridge
7e	Nicholas Aldridge	36	Sean O'Toole	76	Nicholas Aldridge
7g	Nicholas Aldridge	37	Nicholas Aldridge	77	Joost Warsanis
11	Nicholas Aldridge	40 (top)	Nicholas Aldridge	91	Corbis Images
12	Joost Warsanis	42 (top)	Nicholas Aldridge	93	Corbis Images
13	Simon Spiller	44 (top)	NHIL/Nigel Dennis		
14	Mary Evans Picture Library	46 (top)	NHIL/Kelly Walsh		